A strategy to halt and reverse the HIV epidemic among people who inject drugs in Asia and the Pacific 2010-2015

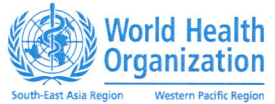 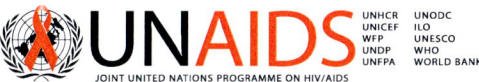 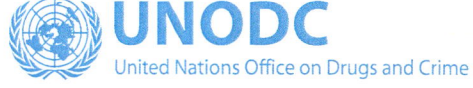

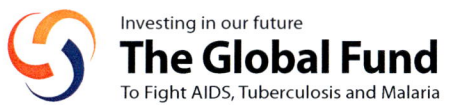 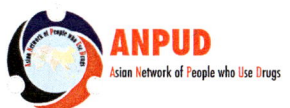

WHO Library Cataloguing in Publication Data

A strategy to halt and reverse the HIV epidemic among people who inject drugs in Asia and the Pacific : 2010–2015

1. HIV infections – prevention and control. 2. Substance abuse, Intravenous – prevention and control. 3. Drug users. 4. Asia and the Pacific.

ISBN 978 92 9061 484 5 (**NLM Classification:** WC 503.6)

© **World Health Organization 2010**

All rights reserved. Publications of the World Health Organization can be obtained from WHO Press, World Health Organization, 20 Avenue Appia, 1211 Geneva 27, Switzerland (tel.: +41 22 791 3264; fax: +41 22 791 4857; e-mail: bookorders@who.int). Requests for permission to reproduce or translate WHO publications – whether for sale or for noncommercial distribution – should be addressed to WHO Press, at the above address (fax: +41 22 791 4806; e-mail: permissions@who.int). For WHO Western Pacific Regional Publications, request for permission to reproduce should be addressed to the Publications Office, World Health Organization, Regional Office for the Western Pacific, P.O. Box 2932, 1000, Manila, Philippines, Fax. No. (632) 521-1036, email: publications@wpro.who.int

The designations employed and the presentation of the material in this publication do not imply the expression of any opinion whatsoever on the part of the World Health Organization concerning the legal status of any country, territory, city or area or of its authorities, or concerning the delimitation of its frontiers or boundaries. Dotted lines on maps represent approximate border lines for which there may not yet be full agreement.

The mention of specific companies or of certain manufacturers' products does not imply that they are endorsed or recommended by the World Health Organization in preference to others of a similar nature that are not mentioned. Errors and omissions excepted, the names of proprietary products are distinguished by initial capital letters.

All reasonable precautions have been taken by the World Health Organization to verify the information contained in this publication. However, the published material is being distributed without warranty of any kind, either expressed or implied. The responsibility for the interpretation and use of the material lies with the reader. In no event shall the World Health Organization be liable for damages arising from its use.

Table of Contents

Acknowledgements	v
Acronyms and abbreviations	vii
Foreword	ix
Introduction	1

A. Situation analysis: HIV, viral hepatitis and drug use in Asia and the Pacific — 3
- A.1 People who inject drugs (PWID) contribute to the overall HIV epidemic — 3
- A.2 Use of amphetamine-type stimulants (ATS) — 4
- A.3 Drug use, HIV and hepatitis C in prisons and detention centres — 5
- A.4 Drug use, HIV and hepatitis C in compulsory centres for drug users — 6

B. Current state of the response to injecting drug use in Asia and the Pacific — 7
- B.1 Legal and policy context — 7
- B.2 Harm reduction services for PWID in Asia and the Pacific — 9

C. Addressing current and emerging priorities in Asia–Pacific, 2010–2015 — 12
- C.1 Addressing the barriers to harm reduction caused by the disconnect between law enforcement and the health sector — 12
- C.2 Scaling up the comprehensive package of interventions for PWUD and PWID — 13
    - *C.2.1 Access to NSP, OST, Condoms and ART* — 14
    - *C.2.2 Condom programmes for PWID and their sexual partners* — 14
    - *C.2.3 Improving access to antiretroviral therapy (ART)* — 15
    - *C.2.4 Addressing the extensive use of compulsory centres for drug users* — 16
    - *C.2.5 Addressing the lack of adequate strategic information* — 18
    - *C.2.6 Addressing the lack of meaningful participation of PWID and PWUD in policy-making and service planning* — 18
- C.3 Addressing emerging priorities in the Asia–Pacific Region — 18
    - *C.3.1 Addressing the lack of testing and treatment for hepatitis B and C* — 18
    - *C.3.2 Addressing the use of amphetamine-type stimulants (ATS)* — 19
    - *C.3.3 Addressing the use of injecting pharmaceuticals* — 20
    - *C.3.4 Addressing emerging drug use and concomitant HIV/AIDS in the Pacific Islands and Territories* — 21
    - *C.3.5 Addressing the lack of attention to drug overdose among out-of-treatment PWID* — 21

D.	**Developing national harm reduction strategies**		**22**
	D.1	Are the proposed interventions cost-effective?	22
	D.2	Can HIV infection be averted through the provision of NSP and OST?	23
	D.3	What is the cost–benefit of averting HIV and hepatitis C?	23
E.	**Goal and objectives of the strategy for Asia and the Pacific**		**25**
	E.1	Development of a national "business" plan	25
		E.1.1 Step 1: Analysis of data on drug use, HIV, hepatitis B and C, and TB: strategic information	*26*
		E.1.2 Step 2: Addressing the barriers to scaling up of harm reduction services	*27*
		E.1.3 Step 3: Setting realistic targets for service provision	*29*
		E.1.4 Step 4: Developing a "costed" national plan (2010–2015)	*31*
F.	**Implementing the regional strategy**		**32**
Annex 1:	**Prevalence of drug use in Asia and the Pacific**		**37**
	Table 1: HIV and hepatitis C prevalence among PWID in selected countries of Asia		*37*
	Table 2: Estimates of PWID in prisons who are HIV positive and have hepatitis B or C		*39*
	Table 3: Clients in compulsory centres for drug users in selected countries		*40*
	Table 4: Amphetamine-type stimulant (ATS) use in selected countries of Asia		*40*
	Table 5: HIV risk behaviours among PWID in selected countries of Asia		*42*
Annex 2:	**Responding to drugs and HIV/AIDS: key international and regional commitments to universal access and harm reduction**		**43**
Annex 3:	**Responding to injecting drug use in selected countries of Asia**		**49**
Annex 4:	**Are NSP and OST effective in reducing high-risk behaviours?**		**53**
Annex 5:	**Organizations in Asia of people who use drugs**		**54**
References			**56**

Acknowledgements

This Regional Strategy to remove the barriers to universal access and harm reduction to halt the spread of HIV and hepatitis C among people who inject drugs in Asia and the Pacific was first proposed by the World Health Organization and has been developed by the United Nations Regional Task Force on Injecting Drug Use and HIV/AIDS for Asia and the Pacific[a] in consultation with Member States in Asia, UN agencies (UNAIDS, UNODC and WHO), major development agencies (World Bank, USAID, AusAID, The Global Fund, the Open Society Institute), academic research institutions, international and national nongovernmental organizations, and civil society networks of people who use drugs and people living with HIV and AIDS.

Consultations were held with many stakeholders during the preparation of the drafts. We would like to express our sincere gratitude to them for their help. Subsequently, a meeting was held in Kuala Lumpur from 7 to 9 December 2009, which was attended by country representatives from Bangladesh, Cambodia, China, India, Indonesia, Lao PDR, Malaysia, Myanmar, Nepal, the Philippines, Thailand and Viet Nam. Special acknowledgement is dedicated to the Swedish International Development Agency (SIDA) and the WHO Regional Office for the Western Pacific for supporting all these activities.

Participants in the process included Dr Robert Ali, Mr Jimmy Dorabjee, Dr Adeeba Kamarulzaman, Dr Suresh Kumar, Mr Dean Lewis, Mr Muhamad Altaf Qamar, Dr Annette Sohn, Ms Tripti Tandon, Dr Alex Wodak, Mr Hadi Yusfian, Ms Robyn Biti, Mr Mauro Guarinieri, Dr Anindya Chatterjee, Mr Lenny Ng Yoon Chong, Ms Nathalie Meyer, Ms Roxanne Saucier, Dr Phauly Tea, Dr Kha Sin Cho, Mr Gray Sattler, Mr Kunal Kishore, Dr Anne Bergenstrom, Dr Cameron Wolf, Dr Aikichi Iwamoto, Mr David Wilson, Ms Nguyen Thi Mai, Dr Massimo Ghidinelli, Dr Fabio Mesquita, Ms Nina Rehn-Mendoza, Mr Graham Shaw, Mr Harpal Singh, Dr David Jacka, Dr Iyanthi Abeyewickreme, Mr Gary Reid, Ms Annette Verster, Dr Mengjie Han, and Dr Nicholas Clark.

Special thanks to Ms Edna Oppenheimer who drafted all the versions of this strategy.

The final draft Regional Strategy for Asia and the Pacific was presented and discussed with participants of the UN Regional Task Force on Injecting Drug Use and HIV/AIDS in Asia and the Pacific meeting in Bangkok from 4 to 5 March 2010. We acknowledge the following for their contribution: Mr Gary Lewis, Mr Fritz Lherisson, Dr Anne Bergenstrom, Dr Fabio Mesquita,

---

[a] The United Nations Regional Task Force on Injecting Drug Use and HIV/AIDS for Asia and the Pacific (UNRTF) was established in 1997 to support the United Nations system to identify priorities and propose strategies, guidelines and options for collaborative activities to respond to HIV/AIDS vulnerability and drug use in the Asia–Pacific Region.

Mr Cho Kah Sin, Ms Sonia Bezziccheri, Mr Ton Smits, Dr Alex Wodak, Mr Tariq Zafar, Mr Luke Samson, Mr Jimmy Dorabjee, Ms Karyn Kaplan, Ms Sekar Wulan Sari, Mr Raj Kumar Raju, Mr Shiba Phurailatpam, Ms Michel Sullivan, Dr Mauro Guarinieri, Dr Swarup Sarkar, Dr Kevin P. Mulvey, Dr Zunyou Wu, Dr Nafsiah Mboi, Dr Ravindra Rao, Mr Ganga Sagar Dhakal, Dr Nawaz Ahmad, Mr Surasak Thanaisawanyangkoon, Ms Chuanpit Choomwattana, Dr Samaruddin, Dr Tasnim Azim, Dr Adeeba Kamarulzaman, Col. Hkam Awng, Dr Suresh Kumar, Ms Margaret Sheehan, Mr Kunal Kishore, Dr Sombat Thanprasertsuk, Ms Edna Oppenheimer, Mr Chris Hagarty and Mr Richard Pearshouse.

Technical editing was done by Dr Bandana Malhotra.

Acronyms and abbreviations

ACDHAP	Asian Consortium on Drug use, HIV, AIDS and Poverty
ANDC	Australian National Council on Drugs
ANPUD	Asian Network of People who Use Drugs
ART	antiretroviral therapy
ASEAN	Association of Southeast Asian Nations
ATS	amphetamine-type stimulants
CSO	civil society organization
DALY	disability-adjusted life-year
ECOSOC	United Nations Economic and Social Council
Global Fund	Global Fund to fight AIDS, Tuberculosis and Malaria
HCV	hepatitis C virus
IBBS	integrated biological and behavioural surveillance
ICAAP	International Congress on AIDS in Asia–Pacific
IEC	information, education and communication
IHRA	International Harm Reduction Association
M&E	monitoring and evaluation
MDG	Millennium Development Goal
MIPUD	meaningful involvement of people who use drugs
MMT	methadone maintenance treatment
N&S	needles and syringes
NGO	nongovernmental organization
NSP	needle and syringe programme
OI	opportunistic infection
OST	opioid substitution therapy
PLHIV	people living with HIV
PWID	people who inject drugs
PWUD	people who use drugs
RAR	rapid assessment and response
RBB	Response Beyond Borders
ROSA	UNODC Regional Office for South Asia

SAARC	South Asian Association for Regional Cooperation
STI	sexually transmitted infection
TAHOD	TREAT Asia from the HIV Observational Database
TB	tuberculosis
TSF	technical support facility
UNAIDS	Joint United Nations Programme on HIV/AIDS
UNGASS	United Nations General Assembly Special Session
UNODC	United Nations Office on Drugs and Crime
UNRTF	United Nations Regional Task Force on Injecting Drug Use and HIV/AIDS for Asia and the Pacific
VCT	voluntary counselling and testing

Foreword

The HIV epidemic continues to evolve in most Asia Pacific countries. Many countries have concentrated epidemics, and some of those epidemics are being driven largely by the unsafe injection of drugs. In the Pacific, more than 10% of cases of HIV infection are related to people who inject drugs in at least two countries. The sexual partners of people who inject drugs are being affected and infected by HIV, and therefore changing the nature of the epidemic in many countries.

The response in the Asia Pacific region to the HIV epidemic among people who inject drugs is varied. There are many needle and syringe programmes, methadone and buprenorphine clinics are becoming increasingly available, and access to antiretroviral therapy for people who use drugs is continuing to increase. But these efforts have not been sufficiently scaled up to halt the spread of HIV. New challenges such as the co-infection with hepatitis C and the increasing use of methamphetamines are impacting the early gains in the response to HIV, jeopardizing further success in the region. In addition, poor promotion of condoms in the current response is facilitating the spread of HIV from people who use drugs to their sexual partners and the population at large.

From 2005 to 2010, WHO Regional Offices for South-East Asia and the Western Pacific have developed a biregional strategy that has served as an advocacy tool bringing science and light to the debate on evidence-based, harm-reduction strategies for the HIV/AIDS support and response. Crucial interventions, such as needle and syringe distribution, methadone and buprenorphine maintenance therapy and access to antiretroviral therapy for people who use drugs, were once issues for debate. Today, they are widely accepted and incorporated in national responses. However, it is now time to enhance the response and further impact the epidemic.

The present document, "A Strategy to Halt and Reverse the HIV Epidemic among People Who Inject Drugs in Asia and the Pacific, 2010–2015" can be a crucial tool. It is a call to action and a road map to ensure that the HIV and hepatitis epidemics among people who use drugs and their sexual partners in the Asia Pacific region will be halted. The strategy is designed to provide a regional framework, and it identifies issues and priorities and provides guidance to countries in the region for developing national strategic responses over the next six years. It shows the important link between halting the HIV epidemic and health and development, and will help countries achieve United Nations Millennium Development Goal 6 that calls for a halt and a reverse in the spread of HIV by 2015.

The strategy reinforces the need for expansion of needle and syringe programmes, wide availability of opioid substitution therapy (methadone and buprenorphine) and universal access to antiretroviral therapy. All of this must occur on a scale that can impact the epidemic. Much needs to be done if we are to achieve universal access. The strategy also addresses new challenges and the responses required to overcome them, including the diagnosis and treatment of the hepatitis C co-infection and the need for evidence-based drug treatment for people who use methamphetamines. All the responses to these challenges should be guided by strategic information and grounded in the meaningful involvement of people who use drugs.

The strategy grew out of intense collaboration and coordination with all key stakeholders in the region. Initiated by the World Health Organization, in coordination with the United Nations Regional Task Force on Injecting Drug Use and HIV/AIDS in Asia and the Pacific, and supported by the community, other development agencies and Member States, the strategy presented here can become a key tool in helping mount the necessary response.

There is a need to improve coordination and work harmoniously as we apply the evidence-based and humanitarian solutions that have been helpful in halting the HIV/ epidemic in other countries over the past 30 years. Members States, nongovernmental organizations, development agencies, other United Nations agencies, universities and people who use drugs must join forces in implementing, monitoring and evaluating the strategy.

The strategy can guide us as we take a great step forward in our efforts towards universal access and the achievement of MDG 6.

Steve Kraus   Gary Lewis

United Nations Regional Task Force
on Injecting Drug Use and HIV/AIDS for Asia and the Pacific

Shin Young-soo, MD, Ph.D.
Regional Director
WHO Western Pacific
Regional Office

Samlee Plianbangchang
Regional Director
WHO South-East Asia
Regional Office

Steve Kraus
Director
UNAIDS Regional Support Team
for Asia and the Pacific

Gary Lewis
Regional Representative
United Nations Office on Drugs and Crime
Regional Centre for East Asia and the Pacific

Mauro Guarinieri
Senior Civil Society Officer, Asia Unit
The Global Fund to Fight AIDS, Tuberculosis
and Malaria

Dean Lewis
Regional Coordinator
Asian Network of People who Use Drugs

Introduction

A regional strategy (2010–2015) for removing the barriers to "universal access"[b] and "harm reduction"[1] to halt the epidemics of HIV and viral hepatitis among and from people who inject drugs (PWID) in Asia and the Pacific was developed by the United Nations Regional Task Force on Injecting Drug Use and HIV/AIDS for Asia and the Pacific. It was developed in pursuit of the sixth Millennium Development Goal (MDG)[2] which is to "Combat HIV/AIDS, malaria and other diseases". Specifically, the targets are to "Halt and begin to reverse the spread of HIV/AIDS among 15–24-year-olds (6.1), increase condom use at high risk sex (6.2) and ensure that those who need it will have universal access to HIV/AIDS treatment including antiretroviral drugs by 2010 (6.5)".[2]

The strategy is a "call for action" designed to provide a practical tool for use by national governments and developing agencies to guide their strategic planning process for the next five years. It provides a framework for harmonizing existing strategies and workplans for harm reduction and universal access.

- The regional strategy is multisectoral, takes a comprehensive approach to drugs, prevention, treatment and care of HIV and hepatitis B and C, and supports evidence- and community-based approaches that aim to reduce the potential harm to health and social functioning from the use of drugs.
- The strategy is inclusive and focuses on people who use drugs (PWUD) and their sexual partners, both of whom are vulnerable to HIV and hepatitis B and C infections.
- The strategy is predicated upon the full participation of civil society, particularly of those who use drugs or are affected directly or indirectly by drugs and related HIV, hepatitis B or C infections.

Although regional drug control and HIV/AIDS prevention policies in Asia and the Pacific are supportive of harm reduction policies and programmes, and endorse the principle of "universal

---

b   Universal access is a global commitment to scale up access to HIV treatment, prevention, care and support. The movement, enshrined in the 2006 UN Political Declaration, is led by countries worldwide with support from UNAIDS and other development partners including civil society.

access" to HIV prevention and treatment, this recognition does not necessarily translate into action or to actions of a significant scale to have an impact on the overall epidemic or on HIV infection levels among PWID. Coverage of essential services varies from country to country and by type of intervention but is overwhelmingly inadequate at present.

The strategy adopts a "right to health" perspective. For PWUD, prevention, treatment and care must be delivered in adequate quantity, be accessible, affordable, of good quality, and provided by well-trained personnel, be culturally, scientifically and medically appropriate, gender sensitive and provided on a voluntary basis[c]. It addresses the fact that well-intentioned commitments to "harm reduction" and "universal access" are not translated into action because of systemic barriers to scaling up interventions, including the different regulatory systems that govern drug use and HIV, as well as considerable financial and human resource gaps. The proposed framework highlights key current and emerging priorities at the regional level and provides information to assist national governments in developing regionally consistent, evidence-based and innovative responses to the problems resulting from injecting drugs, HIV/AIDS and viral hepatitis.

The strategy seeks to improve and enhance national responses by encouraging the sharing of experiences leading to local adaptations of international and regional guidelines and technical briefs. It also encourages the translation of policy statements and declarations of intent into practical, viable and effective national policies and service delivery responses. Finally, the strategy aims to assist major development agencies in Asia and the Pacific to develop their funding strategies to achieve more effective use of limited human and financial resources.

---

c   However, national drug laws in the region are problematic. Most identify drug users as patients as long as they "accept" treatment. All laws have provision for "rehabilitating" drug users - by extended custodial care or "labour therapy".

A. Situation analysis: HIV, viral hepatitis and drug use in Asia and the Pacific

In 2008, an estimated 4.7 million people in Asia were living with HIV (range 3.8–5.5 million) and an estimated 350 000 were newly infected in 2008.[3] In the Pacific Islands and Territories, 29 629 cases were reported in 2008 of people living with HIV (PLHIV) with 5162 new diagnoses of HIV infection . Most of the cases are in Papua New Guinea; over 99% in 2008. The Joint United Nations Programme on HIV/AIDS (UNAIDS) estimates that there are 54 000 PLHIV in the Pacific.[3]

A.1 People who inject drugs (PWID) contribute to the overall HIV epidemic

The sharing of contaminated injecting equipment by PWID is responsible for an increasing number of HIV infections in many countries of Asia. More than half of the world's opiate-using populations are in Asia and one of the four countries with the largest drug-injecting populations in the world is in Asia (China[d]). Furthermore, the prevalence of HIV among PWID is among the highest in any population group. It is estimated that overall, 30% of PWID in South and South-East Asia are HIV positive.[4]

> In South Asia, there are an estimated 569 500 PWID (range 434 000–726 500), of whom between 34 500 and 135 000 are HIV positive (mid-point 74 500).[5]

> In East and South-East Asia, there are an estimated 3 957 500 PWID (range 3 043 500–4 913 00) and about 313 000–1 251 500 (mid-point 661 000) are HIV infected.[5]

> In the Pacific Islands and Territories, there are an estimated 14 500–25 000 PWID (mid-point 19 500), of whom an estimated 1.37% are HIV positive (<250–500).[5]

In many countries of Asia, PWID contribute disproportionally to the total number of people who are HIV positive. Thus, for example, in China in 2007, 29.9% of new infections were traced back to PWID[6] and an analysis of the cumulative reported HIV cases in China (2008) found that 38.5% of cases could be traced back to injection drug use.[7] In Indonesia, 46% of infections in 2007 were attributed to injecting drug use[8] and 57% of new infections in 2008 in Malaysia.[9] In Bangladesh, PWID accounted for almost 9 out of 10 HIV-positive cases found in the 2006 serosurveillance survey[10] and, in some islands of the Pacific, despite the fact that the overall

---

d   The other three are Brazil, USA and the Russian Federation.

prevalence of injecting drug use is low, it significantly contributes to HIV prevalence. Excluding Papua New Guinea, PWID represented 6.3% of total HIV infections in the Pacific region and in some islands. For example, in French Polynesia, PWID account for 11.7% and in New Caledonia 10.1% of cumulative HIV cases on the island.[11] It is impossible to predict future trends in drug consumption because of the volatility of the drug markets and consumption patterns.

HIV/AIDS high-risk behaviours among PWID and PWUD: There is ample anecdotal evidence that PWID in Asia and the Pacific continue to engage in high-risk behaviours both in the community and in closed centres. Official country reports to the United Nations in pursuit of the Declaration of Commitment on HIV/AIDS, which was adopted by the General Assembly in June 2001, are not comprehensive and data are often based on small selected samples. However, the following research findings illustrate the diversity in the region.

- Self-reported use of unsterile injecting equipment varied from 71% in one state in India (Sikkim) to 12% in Kolkata, India, and from 7% of PWID in Nepal to 34% of male and 74% of females in Bangladesh.[12]

- Practising safe sex: The risk for acquiring HIV infection from unsafe sex affects both PWUD and their partners. It cannot be assumed that when PWID practise safe injecting they also practise safe sex. Reported condom use during last sex is variable, ranging from 31% in Pakistan, 34% in Indonesia, 43% in Bangladesh, and from 44% to 100% in India.[12]

- In the Pacific Islands and Territories, the connections between alcohol, drugs, unsafe sex (including decreased condom use) and vulnerability to HIV are evident across the region. Recent surveys have found that around a third of all young people used alcohol and drugs before their last sexual encounter.[11]

- A number of studies in South Asia provide additional confirmatory information that spouses and sexual partners of men who inject drugs are at high risk for HIV.[11]

Note: Table 1 in Annex 1 provides information about injecting drug use, HIV and hepatitis C prevalence among PWID in Asia and the Pacific.

A.2 Use of amphetamine-type stimulants (ATS)

The most recent global estimates of the use of amphetamine-type stimulants (ATS) exceed that of heroin and cocaine use.[13] It has been estimated that, in 2007, between 4.6 million and 20.6 million people in East and South-East Asia used ATS and between 2 250 000 and 5 950 00 were ecstasy users.[5]

ATS is often used orally, though crystal methamphetamine is increasingly being injected. However, ATS users are vulnerable to HIV whether or not they inject. When they do not inject, they are at risk for infection from unsafe sex practised when intoxicated with ATS. For those who do turn to injecting, their risks of becoming infected through sharing of infected injecting equipment are similar to that of other PWID, regardless of the substance injected.

There are indications of increasing demand for methamphetamine in Thailand, which may have wide implications for neighbouring countries, for example, increased trafficking and the risk of clandestine laboratory operations being established, or increased use in the border areas of Lao PDR and Cambodia. Viet Nam may emerge as a vulnerable market as methamphetamine manufacturers seek to diversify away from their reliance on the Thai market. In addition, the changing political situation in Myanmar in 2009 might serve as a push factor for illicit drugs and relocation of clandestine manufacturing sites across its borders.

In South Asia, the United Nations Office on Drugs and Crime (UNODC) Regional ATS report[13] suggests that although data are limited, "the region is attractive to organized crime groups seeking to manufacture ATS, as a result of a large licit industry for production of ATS precursor chemicals. In addition, there is limited awareness of, and experience with ATS, and a potentially large market. The law enforcement effort focuses primarily on traditional drugs of trafficking and use, such as heroin, cannabis and pharmaceutical preparations".

In the Pacific Islands and Territories,[5] the absence of formal surveillance systems, both nationally and regionally, makes accurate assessments difficult. With the exception of Guam and the Commonwealth of Northern Mariana Islands, which have established methamphetamine markets,[14] the evidence for ATS use has been limited. There are emerging reports of methamphetamine use in the States and Territories of American Samoa, French Polynesia, Fiji, Palau, Papua New Guinea, Samoa and Vanuatu.[23]

Overall, the number of countries in Asia and the Pacific reporting methamphetamine as their primary drug of use (in either pill or crystalline form) have remained largely the same over the past four years. However, methamphetamine has rapidly become more prominent in some countries, which now rank it as the second most common drug.[13] The lack of research and surveillance causes concern that everywhere new patterns and trends in drug use may emerge and become entrenched before effective prevention and treatment resources can be mobilized.

Note: Table 4 in Annex 1 provides information on ATS use in countries in Asia

A.3 Drug use, HIV and hepatitis C in prisons and detention centres

Many countries in Asia have a "zero tolerance" to drug use and drug trafficking, resulting in a stringent application of narcotic legislation and a large prison population of PWUD or ex-users. Routinely, possession of certain quantities of drugs is deemed to signify trafficking – although all too often PWUD are also traffickers, selling drugs to finance their drug use.[15]

Malaysia reported that that 33% of prisoners are incarcerated for drug-related offences and 60% for drug-related crimes.[16] In Pakistan, according to official data in 2009, 3630 PWUD were incarcerated (including six female drug users).[e] It is estimated that 63% of prisoners in India had "ever" used drugs but it is unclear what they used or when. Likewise, 86% of prisoners in Sri Lanka had used drugs at some time and 37% of prisoners in Viet Nam were PWID. In some countries such as Indonesia, there are narcotic prisons to house, treat and rehabilitate PWUD but some drug offenders/users are found in general prisons and detention centres. In addition, some countries in Asia also have a system of administrative detention and re-education through labour, in which many PWUD are incarcerated (e.g. Viet Nam and China).

Information about prisoner health including data on the prevalence of HIV, hepatitis C, sexually transmitted infections (STIs) and opportunistic infections (OIs) is sketchy. Health budgets for the prison services are uniformly low. In some countries, HIV prevalence in prison is higher than that in the community.[16] HIV prevalence among prisoners in Indonesia is estimated at 22% (2002)[17] and in Cambodia prevalence is estimated to be 3.1%.[18] HIV among prisoners with a history of drug use is rarely recorded separately so data are scant (0.8% among PWID prisoners in India and 0.28% among PWID prisoners in Viet Nam).[f]

Note: For additional data on prison populations in countries in Asia and the Pacific, see Table 2 in Annex 1.

A.4   Drug use, HIV and hepatitis C in compulsory centres for drug users

Compulsory centres for drug users to which PWUD are committed are also high-risk environments for HIV and hepatitis C transmission. However, there is a dearth of reliable data and it is not always clear whether residents arrived in these centres already infected or whether they became infected in the centres. Many do not know their HIV or hepatitis C status. As in prisons, there is anecdotal evidence of unsterile drug use and of unsafe sexual behaviours in these settings. For example, high rates of incarceration of young methamphetamine users in Thailand have been associated with a range of HIV and hepatitis C risk behaviours, including injecting and tattooing.[19] A study in six Vietnamese 06 centres found HIV prevalence ranging from 30% to 35[20] and in China, the national HIV prevalence in the Rehabilitation through Labour Centres was 5%.[21]

Note: See table 3 in Annex 1 for information about compulsory centres for drug users in the region.

---

e   Personal communication from UNODC Islamabad, Pakistan

f   UNODC unpublished data, 2009

B. Current state of the response to injecting drug use in Asia and the Pacific

B.1 Legal and policy context

A summary of key international commitments to universal access and harm reduction

A number of international commitments and frameworks adopt harm reduction principles for the implementation of HIV and harm reduction activities, including the following:

- Declaration of Commitment on HIV/AIDS by the United Nations General Assembly 26th Special Session (UNGASS), 27 June 2001;[21]
- Resolution of the United Nations General Assembly High-level Meeting on HIV/AIDS;[22]
- Universal access for PWUD to all HIV and AIDS treatment is articulated in the WHO/UNAIDS Care and treatment for people who inject drugs in Asia and the Pacific: an essential practice guide[23]
- WHO, UNODC, UNAIDS Technical guide for target setting for HIV prevention, treatment and care for injecting drug users (2009)[24]
- UNAIDS, the 24th Programme Coordinating Board (PCB) (2009)[25]
- UNAIDS outcome framework 2009–2011[26]
- United Nations Economic and Social Council: Commission on Narcotic Drugs. Report on the 52nd session (14 March 2008 and 11–20 March 2009). New York, Official Records 2009, Suppl. No 8 (E/2009/28).[27]
- The Human Rights Council Resolutions: A/HRC/12/L.23[28] on access to medicines in the context of the right to the highest attainable standard of health, and A/HRC/12/L.24 on the protection of human rights in the context of HIV/AIDS.[29]

All international policy statements and commitments are unanimous in endorsing and promoting comprehensive harm reduction services; ensuring that these services are accessible, affordable and equitable; and providing prevention, treatment and care services for all people including PWUD and PWID by 2010. UNAIDS is charged with working with its co-sponsors to coordinate this effort.

The 2006 UN High-Level Meeting on AIDS provided guidance to countries about developing appropriate indicators to measure progress towards universal access and requested Member States to report regularly on the state of the HIV and AIDS epidemic in their countries.[22] However, a recent review of the UNAIDS Programme Coordinating Board (2009) noted that a "gap" still existed in the international and national response to PWUD.[25] The Board, therefore, recommended that UNAIDS' co-sponsors support the development of comprehensive models targeting PWUD and supporting national authorities to align their policies and improve the collection of strategic information. Subsequently, the UNAIDS Outcome Framework[26] identified nine interlinked priorities, which include the following:

- "Reducing sexual transmission of HIV",
- "Protecting drug users from become infected with HIV",
- "Removing punitive laws, policies and practices, stigma and discrimination that block effective responses to AIDS", and
- "Ensuring that the people living with HIV (PLHIV) receive treatment".

Universal access must be more than a "wish list" and should be implemented through a concrete process of identifying critical barriers to scaling up, and making plans to address these issues. Universal access encompasses the principles of equality, sustainability, comprehensiveness, accessibility and sustainability. Thus:[24]

- Services should be physically accessible and available including in prisons and other closed settings.
- Services must be affordable.
- Services must be equitable and non-discriminatory with no exclusion criteria, except on medical grounds.
- Treatment should not be rationed: supply should be determined by need and not limited by cost or other considerations.
- Access should not be determined by sociodemographic factors such as age, sex/gender, sexual orientation and sexual behaviour, citizenship, race/ethnicity, asylum-seeking, refugee status, employment status and profession (including sex work).
- All interventions should be offered voluntarily in an enabling environment created by supportive legislation, policies and strategies.

Legal and policy context: a summary of key regional commitments to universal access and harm reduction

A number of regional commitments and frameworks adopt harm reduction principles for the implementation of HIV and harm reduction activities, including the following:

- Association of Southeast Asian Nations (ASEAN) commitments on HIV and AIDS[30,31]
- The Commission on AIDS in Asia (2008): Redefining AIDS in Asia: crafting an effective response[32]
- The UNODC Regional Programme Framework for East Asia and the Pacific (2009–2012)[33] and Regional Programme for South Asia (2008–2011).[34]

Following on the pursuit of a drug-free ASEAN of 2000, the commitments on HIV and AIDS (2007–08)[30] reflect a commitment in ASEAN countries to focus efforts on providing services to PWUD to prevent HIV infection. This is reflected in the workplan programme on HIV and AIDS III (2006–2010)[35] in which the need is emphasized to protect the health of PWID, their partners, families and communities, by facilitating all effective means (including access to clean needles and syringes) to prevent the spread of bloodborne viruses including HIV.

The Commission on AIDS in Asia notes, however, that of the 11 countries in Asia with drug-related HIV epidemics, none offers comprehensive harm reduction services for PWUD.[32]

UNODC in South and South-East Asia aims to address the low coverage, poor strategic information and little mainstreaming of HIV services for PWUD. A further major objective of the regional programmes is to harmonize the public health and law enforcement perspective on harm reduction. Thus, UNODC in South Asia plans to encourage a policy dialogue between the two sectors and will endeavour to move stakeholders towards a position where care can be provided in an evidence-based manner and in consonance with what the law will allow.[34]

To summarize:

Harm reduction is now generally accepted by the majority of countries in the region and favourably acknowledged in key health and AIDS policy documents. Nevertheless, the overwhelming approach to injecting drug use is compulsory incarceration in "treatment" institutions for lengthy periods of time. The disconnection between the public health and judicial and extra judicial approaches to drug use remains a critical barrier to successful implementation of harm reduction.

Note: See Annex 2 for an expanded account of the global and regional legal and policy situation.

B.2   Harm reduction services for PWID in Asia and the Pacific

Harm reduction services in the community: needle and syringe programmes and opioid substitution therapy

A regional analysis of national policies on harm reduction in Asia and the Pacific reported by the International Harm Reduction Association (IHRA) (2008)[18] indicates that overall, countries are committed to providing comprehensive harm reduction interventions. Thirteen countries and territories have domestic policies on drugs or HIV that explicitly include harm reduction. These are: Afghanistan, Bangladesh, Cambodia, China and Hong Kong, India, Indonesia, Lao PDR, Myanmar, Nepal, Pakistan and Viet Nam. All Asian countries have national HIV plans,[9] several of which include harm reduction, injecting drug use and human rights.

---

g   Bangladesh, Cambodia, India, Indonesia, Lao PDR, Nepal, Pakistan and Sri Lanka

For those countries without explicit policies that include harm reduction, there are indications that the situation is due to change. For example, in the Philippines, a harm reduction policy is currently being developed and in Pakistan the government is supportive of harm reduction activities that are implemented by civil society. In Thailand, the national AIDS plan for 2007–2011[36] aims to improve access to HIV prevention, treatment and care for both PWUD and prisoners.

However, this widespread acceptance (generally in HIV/AIDS strategic documents) does not necessarily translate into action. Not only is the service coverage very low, but in most countries of the region there is a continuing disconnect between the approach to PWUD by law enforcement authorities and the public health sector.

Most countries have some targeted services in place to prevent HIV among PWID but in none of them is the coverage of services adequate. The summary table (Table 1, Annex 3) is designed to demonstrate that the coverage of needle and syringe programmes (NSP) and opioid substitution therapy (OST) for PWID is overwhelmingly inadequate. Even in countries where PWID are disproportionately affected by HIV, the numbers being treated with antiretroviral therapy (ART) is believed to be low (current or previous history of drug injecting is not routinely recorded, but anecdotal information from PWUD suggests that in general only ex-users are being treated with ART, with the possible exception of PWUD on methadone treatment, in some countries).

Note: See Tables 1 and 2 in Annex 3 for summary information about NSP and OST services in Asia and the Pacific.

HIV/AIDS prevention services for prisoners and those in detention centres in Asia and the Pacific

Effective policies to prevent HIV in prisons and other correctional institutions are hampered by the denial of the existence of factors that contribute to the spread of HIV, tuberculosis (TB) and other infections, coupled with a chronic lack of resources. Prisons in the region are characterized by overcrowding, drug use, unsafe sex, a lack of adequate protection and safety for young inmates and women, and prevailing corruption.[37] Even though basic health-care services are limited, voluntary counselling and testing (VCT) for HIV and ART is available in some prisons (e.g. in Indonesia, India, Myanmar and Thailand) but, overall, these services are not to scale and not applied universally. Some prisons and detention centres offer minimal information, education and communication (IEC) to inmates, generally provided by nongovernmental organizations (NGOs), but these vary in both quality and intensity. A few provide condoms and/or disinfecting substances to enable cleaning of needles and syringes.

Indonesia was the first country in Asia to endorse an HIV/AIDS strategy for prisons and detention centres[38] and introduced methadone maintenance treatment (MMT) targeting PWID in three prisons, which was provided to a total of 70 prisoners.[h] In Malaysia, there are 36 937 prisoners of whom 33% are drug offenders and 60% are in prison for drug-related crimes. Four per cent are HIV positive. Malaysia has OST programmes in 11 prisons, supported by UNODC, which provides MMT to approximately 300 pre-release prisoners.[15]

In South Asia (Bangladesh, India, Maldives, Nepal and Sri Lanka), 26 prison interventions have been supported by UNODC. Behaviour change education is provided, which aims to empower prisoners to engage in positive health behaviours with regard to drugs and HIV during incarceration and after release. Through these interventions, the project has reached out to 26 000 prisoners and trained 400 master trainers. Only one prison has a pilot OST programme providing buprenorphine to approximately 60 prisoners. In Pakistan a project in nine jails in Sind province (April 2004–December 2009) provided peer education to 30 502 inmates and VCT was conducted with 11 570 prisoners. Two hundred thirty-five HIV infections were detected, and care and support were provided to 214. IEC material (93 237 items) and condoms (20 325) were distributed, and ART was provided to 31 prisoners.[i]

Needle and syringe programmes are unavailable in Asian prisons.

To summarize:

Harm reduction services in the community, prisons or in other drug treatment facilities are, with few exceptions, not provided "to scale", a necessary prerequisite for halting and averting the epidemics of HIV and hepatitis. Coverage of the essential package of services for PWUD in Asia remains unacceptably low. Furthermore, there is evidence that certain vulnerable groups of PWUD, e.g. out-of-school or unemployed youth, male and female sex workers, transgender people, minority populations, refugees and other displaced people[39,40] are frequently ignored when services are designed and planned.

---

h   Data received from MoH Indonesia. Personal communication, February 2010

i   Information from Sukkur Blood and Drugs Donating Society (SBDDS) 2010 Service Delivery Project for the Prevention of HIV/AIDS for jail inmates in Sindh province

C. Addressing current and emerging priorities in Asia–Pacific, 2010–2015

In order to achieve universal access and provide harm reduction services, a number of current and emerging priorities have to be addressed.

C.1 Addressing the barriers to harm reduction caused by the disconnect between law enforcement and the health sector

Below is a brief analysis of the reasons why the above are considered priorities in the region. A summary of the evidence is also presented.

In all countries of the region, there are several regulatory drug and HIV systems, which operate side by side, and a number of different legal entities concerned with drug control and health issues. At the moment, many countries provide harm reduction services (particularly NSP) despite legal ambiguities. Indeed, the problems encountered often lie in the ad hoc interpretation and application of the law by enforcement officials.

There seem to be two major areas of ambiguity, which inhibit the scale up of harm reduction services.[41,42]

- The provision of sterile needles constitutes "abetment" or "facilitation" of illicit consumption. The wording of this clause differs from country to country but the net result is the same. Examples include the following:

    - In Cambodia, the provision of needles and syringes may be interpreted as "intentional facilitation" and inciting "unlawful use".[j,42] The licensing of NSP by the National Authority for Combating Drugs is slow and NGOs providing NSP report considerable "harassment" by local police.[k]
    - In Bangladesh, possession of injecting paraphernalia is not an offence but distribution of sterile needles may amount to abetment of illicit use, punishable with three to fifteen

---

j   UN agencies have been advocating for the introduction of articles on harm reduction, health services and drug treatment into the new drug law.

k   Personal communication from NGO workers (2010)

years imprisonment and a fine. Organizations that let premises to NGOs to run NSP can be prosecuted.

- In India, although the possession of injecting equipment is not illegal, the provision of sterile injecting equipment to a PWID may amount to aiding and abetting the offence of unlawful consumption of drugs.
- In Lao PDR, supplying sterile injection equipment to PWID is an offence.
- In Malaysia, carrying injecting equipment with traces of drugs creates a presumption of possession.
- In Myanmar, the provision of needles and syringes (N&S) is prohibited (but it does not deter NGOs and the UN from operating NSP).
- In Nepal, the distribution of N&S may be construed as aiding and abetting drug use.
- In Pakistan, supplying injecting equipment to a PWUD may be punishable as abetment.
- In the Philippines, possession of injecting material is permitted only to medical practitioners.
- In Thailand, NSP are seen as instigating another person to use drugs and are prohibited.

- Dispensing methadone amounts to an offence where it is a prohibited drug and oral substitution lacks a legal basis in countries where drug treatment is statutorily defined as abstinence.
  - In several countries of the region, the legal basis for OST is compromised, e.g. in Bangladesh where methadaone is a prohibited drug, and in India where it is still unclear whether OST is for medical use or detoxification, and where methadone is not legally available (although buprenorphine is). In Lao PDR, the status of methadone and buprenorphine for OST is unclear. In Pakistan, any oral substitution may be in contravention of the law, unless permitted within the exception of supply for medical treatment. In the Philippines, methadone is a prohibited drug.

The implications of this disharmony are twofold:
- PWUD and PWID are criminalized, discouraging health-seeking behaviour, and
- Reluctance on the part of some national governments to own and scale up harm reduction services.

It will thus be crucial in the next five years to work towards a reconciliation of the different regulatory systems and diverse objectives that govern existing approaches to drug control so that the lawful expansion of harm reduction services is not impeded.

C.2   Scaling up the comprehensive package of interventions for PWUD and PWID

As has been noted above in the analysis of the state of the harm reduction, much needs to be done to scale up services, in order to achieve the goal of halting the epidemics of HIV and viral hepatitis. It is important that all interventions are evidence- and community based.

The WHO, UNODC, UNAIDS Technical guide for target setting[24] spells out what the UNAIDS and its co-sponsors understand by "comprehensive" prevention, treatment and care programmes for PWID. The package comprises nine essential interventions:

1. NSP
2. OST and other drug dependence treatment
3. ART
4. HIV testing and counselling
5. Condom programmes for PWID and their sexual partners
6. Prevention and treatment of STIs
7. Targeted IEC for PWID and their sexual partners
8. Vaccination for, and diagnosis and treatment of, viral hepatitis
9. Prevention, diagnosis and treatment of TB.

Just four of the above essential interventions are specifically directed at PWUD (1, 2, 6, 7). The others should be provided as part of national HIV and AIDS strategies. However, access to ART is also discussed below because it remains problematic for PWUD. In addition, although not specifically noted in the "essential package", it should be remembered that PWUD and PWID among populations groups such as sex workers, transgender people, migrants, refugees, internally displaced people have special needs and very specific difficulties in accessing services.

C.2.1 Access to NSP, OST, Condoms and ART

These nine interventions are included in the comprehensive package because they have the greatest impact on HIV prevention and treatment. While each of these separate interventions is useful in addressing HIV prevention and care among PWID, it is important to recognize that they form part of a package and have the greatest beneficial impact when delivered together. These interventions are also appropriate for prisons. The principle of equivalency of care demands that prisoners are entitled, without discrimination, to the same standard of health care that is found in the outside community, including preventive measures and ART. In countries with limited resources, is it advised that at least five of the nine interventions – NSP, OST, Condoms, HIV testing and counselling and ART – be implemented.[43] It should also be noted that apart from the first two, the other interventions are (or should be) routinely delivered as part of the HIV and AIDS strategic plans.

The lack of all health services in prisons and detention centres needs special consideration. Here, it is not just PWUD who are at risk for infectious diseases, but all prisoners.

C.2.2 Condom programmes for PWID and their sexual partners

There is evidence of unsafe sexual practices among PWID, as seen by HIV infection among non-injecting partners of PWID. Overall, condoms were used less frequently with regular partners (e.g. wives) than with casual partners.[44] Several studies in South Asia have examined condom use by PWID:

Study	Sample	Condom used at last sex	Partners engaged in sex work
Rapid situation and response assessment in South Asia (2008)[45]	4612 regular female partners of PWID	10.3% in Bangladesh, 21.5% in India, 36.5% in Nepal and 11.7% in Sri Lanka	22.8% in Bangladesh, 7.5% in India, 13.7% in Nepal and 10.5% in Sri Lanka
The hidden truth, a study of HIV vulnerability, risk factors and prevalence[46]	459 couples in Pakistan	20% (5–15% of wives of those who were HIV positive were infected)	No information
Transmission of HIV from PWID to their wives in India[47]	160 couples recruited between 1996 and 1997	45% of wives were HIV positive	The male subjects were not tested but in Manipur where the study took place, 80% of PWID are HIV positive
Rapid situation assessment of HIV prevalence and risk factors among PWID in four cities in the Punjab[44]	Mapping of street-based PWUD: M. Bahauddin 713–928, in Rawalpindi 348–451, in Gujranwala 466–607 and 267–460 in Sheikhupura	Condom with regular partner NEVER; 73% in M. Bahauddin, 62% in Rawalpindi, 57% in Gujranwala and 75% in Sheikhupura	No information
Rapid situation assessment in Pakistan[48]	169 women – regular sex partners of 715 PWID	20.7%	No information

As is evident from the studies above, sexual partners are at high risk for HIV and it is important to ensure that adequate resources are made available for prevention, treatment and care of these highly vulnerable women. Basic services include IEC for PWID and their partners, as well as ready access to condoms. It will be necessary to overcome the reluctance of PWUD to use condom with regular partners.

C.2.3 Improving access to antiretroviral therapy (ART)

In East, South and South-East Asia, 565 000 (520 000–610 000) people were receiving ART at the end of 2008. This represents a regional increase of 35% in one year and an eightfold increase over the 70 000 (52 000–88 000) people receiving treatment at the end of 2003.[12] Access to ART for PWUD and PWID is difficult to monitor because drug use status is not routinely recorded in

AIDS services. Where information is gathered, it is apparent that although in some countries PWUD and PWID constitute the largest number of PLHIV, the number of current HIV-positive PWUD receiving ART remains disproportionately low. For example, in Malaysia, PWID comprise 75% of all HIV cases, and only 5% of those receiving ART, and although around 50% of PWUD in Indonesia are HIV positive, the percentage of those on ART is as low as 3%.[8] In China, there are 67 900 people receiving ART of whom 16% are PWUD.[49] Some of the barriers to ART were identified by the APN+ study (2009).[l,50]

> **The sample:** 945 PWID living with HIV were recruited to the study: 200 from China, 155 from India, 263 from Indonesia, 86 from Myanmar, 100 from Nepal and 100 from Viet Nam.
>
> **Results:** more than half (59%) reported being in need of ART yet not receiving treatment.
> Of the women, 1/3 who were currently on ART considered access to ART services either "difficult" or "very difficult".
>
> **Barriers to treatment included:** a lack of knowledge about ART, no ART in the area, fear of side-effects and drug interactions, interactions between active drug use and antiretroviral medication, distance to ART facilities, unfriendly provider attitude and denial of health services.

Contrary to initial expectations by health-care personnel, ART has been successfully provided for PWID. A large number of patients who were offered ART have been retained in and assisted by treatment, and outcomes have been comparable with those of non-drug-using patients. Furthermore, combining HIV/AIDS care with substance dependence treatment services (including OST) has been particularly successful.[23]

To sum up, several systemic difficulties inhibit equitable access to ART for PWUD and PWID. These include, first and foremost, the need to dispel the misconceptions about the impact of drug use on adherence to ART, lack of OST, which has the potential to maximize adherence, and insufficient information targeted at PWUD about the treatment and its benefits. It is also evident that stigma and discrimination against PWID is rife in health-care settings.

C.2.4 Addressing the extensive use of compulsory centres for drug users

Compulsory centres for drug users are a common approach to "treatment" of drug users in the region, despite coming under increased scrutiny and criticism from UN agencies, development agencies and human rights organizations.[51,52] This approach is widely used by Cambodia, China, Lao PDR, Malaysia, Myanmar, Thailand and Viet Nam. Some countries, e.g. Lao PDR, Thailand and Viet Nam, are continuing to increase the number and capacity of the centres. By 2009, Lao PDR had increased the number of such centres to nine while Thailand now has 84 and planned to build 14 more in 2009. In Viet Nam, between 50 000 and 100 000 people were interned in

---

l APN+ is a regional network of PLHIV, which represents individuals and groups throughout the Asia–Pacific region and is an organization run by, and for, PLHIV.

the 05'06' "education and social labour centres" whose numbers have risen to 109.[m] Some countries have begun to turn away from this approach, notably China and Malaysia.[m]

A key feature of these institutions is the limitation of personal freedom. The centres contravene international human rights law which seeks to ensure the right to due process before incarceration. Many PWUD (and some who do not even use drugs but are rounded up in the street), including minors, are routinely brought in to the centres by the police or are incarcerated at the behest of their families, who can leave their relatives in the centres for an indeterminate period of time. UNODC/WHO[53] have observed that the functioning of the centres is rarely implemented in a way that is consistent with international standards and is not evidence based. The report recommends that UNODC and WHO take specific steps to disseminate current evidence on drug dependence and notes that:

> *"As any medical procedure, in general conditions drug dependence treatment, be it psychosocial or pharmacological, should not be forced on patients.... A patient is entitled to reject treatment and choose the penal sanctions instead... treatment is offered as an alternative to incarceration or other penal sanctions, but not imposed without consent.... Neither detention nor forced labour has been recognised by science as a treatment for drug use disorders."*

UNODC and WHO propose that in order for drug dependence services to reach the maximum number of individuals in need and to be effective in halting and reversing the HIV/AIDS epidemic among PWID, the best way is to establish broad community-based[n] services that can serve individuals in their own communities. They should offer pragmatic, effective services and use internationally approved guidelines and methodologies.

See Table 3 in Annex 1 for additional information on centres for compulsory drug treatment in Asia.

---

m   UNODC/United Nations Regional Task Force on Injecting Drug Use and HIV/AIDS in Asia and the Pacific. Working Group on CDTCs. Briefing Note Agenda Item 10. Compulsory treatment centres in East Asia. Bangkok, Thailand, July 2009 (not officially published)

n   Community-based drug treatment refers specifically to an integrated model of treatment in the community. It includes services from detoxification through to aftercare and also involves the coordination of any number of non-specialist services that are needed to meet clients' needs. Research compiled by UNODC suggests that the goals of community-based treatment are:

  • To encourage behaviour change directly in the community

  • To actively involve local organizations, community members and target populations in the establishment of an integrated network of community-based services in a manner that is empowering.

  A key focus of community-based treatment is on reaching people who are affected by the harms of substance abuse with limited access to services.

C.2.5 Addressing the lack of adequate strategic information

As is clear from the tables in Annexes 1 and 3, reliable information is not easily available about the extent of drug use, types of substances used, prevalence of injecting drug use, levels of high-risk behaviours, geographical locations of drug use, and drug use, HIV and hepatitis in the community, prisons and forced "treatment" centres. For planning to be effective and properly targeted, strategic information is essential.

In order to achieve this, attention must be given to training for data gathering, analysis and research, and to ensuring sufficient financial allocation for this to take place.

C.2.6 Addressing the lack of meaningful participation of PWID and PWUD in policy-making and service planning

"Nothing about us without us" – this rallying cry was formulated by the Canadian HIV/AIDS Legal Network in partnership with PWUD groups in Vancouver in 2005. Their objectives are to call on governments, bilateral and multilateral organizations, civil society organizations (CSOs) and the general public to support them in

> *"Empowering our communities to advocate and protect our rights and to facilitate meaningful participation in decision-making on issues affecting us";*

and for

> *"Supporting, strengthening and encouraging the development of organizations for people who use drugs in communities/countries where they do not exist". And…(to) challenge existing oppressive drug laws, policies and programmes and work with government and our constituents to formulate evidence-based drug policies that respect human rights and dignity of people who use drugs."*

This strategy for Asia and the Pacific supports the Asian Network of People who Use Drugs (ANPUD) and will provide support for the expansion of the regional network, and the seeding and development of active national networks.

Note: For more on the development of Response Beyond Borders and ANPUD, see Annex 5.

C.3 Addressing emerging priorities in the Asia–Pacific Region

C.3.1 Addressing the lack of testing and treatment for hepatitis B and C

An article in the *Medical Journal of Australia* in 1997 entitled "Waiting for the grim reaper"[54] warned of a potential hepatitis C epidemic and argued for the need to raise awareness of the dangers and seriousness of this disease. Indeed, data published by the WHO in 1999[55] revealed that Asian countries have some of the highest national hepatitis C virus (HCV) prevalence rates in the world. By 2007, the prevalence of hepatitis C in South-East Asia was estimated at 2.15%, representing 25 million people living with HCV.[56] Data on the prevalence of hepatitis C among PWID in the region are incomplete (see data in Annex 1) and is estimated to be <5% but available data indicate that coinfections of HIV and hepatitis C among PWUD in some countries are extremely high (50–100%, e.g. in the Philippines, Bangladesh, Viet Nam[57]). A recent study of PWUD in Manipur[58] where HCV testing was provided to 70 former and current PWID found that around 70–80% of the PWID who took part were coinfected with HIV and none was receiving treatment for hepatitis. In the APN+ study[50] referred to above, around two third of PWID knew that HIV-positive people are more likely to be coinfected with hepatitis but less than half had been tested for the virus. The results indicated that nearly 6% of those who had been tested and received their test results were positive for both HIV and HCV. Here also, none of them were receiving treatment.

Consequences: In a meeting of CSOs at the International Congress on AIDS in Asia–Pacific (ICAAP) meeting in Bali (2009), the refusal to recognize and treat HIV–hepatitis C coinfections was said to have dampened the optimism for universal access. The impact of coinfection is serious. In the short term, it leads to poorer treatment outcomes on ART, "flares" of disease during immune reconstitution, less tolerance of treatment interruptions and a reduced response to hepatitis treatment. In the long term, it increases the risk of disease progression, and can result in higher hepatitis viral loads, cirrhosis, hepatocellular carcinoma and death.[59]

No vaccine is available for the prevention of hepatitis C. Treatment consists of pegylated interferon plus ribavirin for 24 or 48 weeks. The response is a suppressed HCV RNA viral load of 40–90% after 48 weeks' treatment. However, as with ARV medication a decade ago, the high cost of hepatitis C treatment regimens is a major barrier to providing treatment. Estimates of the total cost are difficult because they vary across countries (e.g. treatment costs in the United Kingdom in 2007 was £11 000).

Strong advocacy is needed in Asia and the Pacific to reduce the cost of medicines, increase education on the issue of hepatitis C, and train health providers and other relevant services to provide social and emotional support to people undertaking treatment of hepatitis C.

C.3.2 Addressing the use of amphetamine-type stimulants (ATS)

The case for addressing the lack of services and evidence-based treatment for ATS users in Asia and the Pacific has been made earlier. Fifty-five per cent of the world's total number of ATS users is in Asia[60] and although the majority are oral users, predicting future drug use patterns is impossible. There is evidence of increasing use of crystal methamphetamine by injection. Meanwhile, there is irrefutable evidence that ATS users engage in high-risk sexual behaviours, hence the importance of addressing this emerging issue in the next five years.[61]

The lack of evidence-based services for ATS users in Asia and the Pacific is serious and has resulted in tens of thousands being incarcerated in compulsory centres for drug users and other forms of detention facilities. In order to ensure a rights- and evidence-based approach, it will be important to urgently develop an evidence base and effective voluntary treatment services for ATS users. Such evidence as exists suggests that these should be rooted in a public health approach, and be community based, flexible and multifocused. These include "stepped care" and risk reduction approaches developed and suitable for countries in Asia and the Pacific, and geared towards the specific needs of ATS users.

C.3.3 Addressing the use of injecting pharmaceuticals

The goal of providing comprehensive harm reduction services and universal access to PWUD is generally confined to those who use "illegal" drugs such as opioids or ATS. The harmful use of pharmaceutical drugs which are "legal drugs" and easily available in unregulated pharmacies in many countries of Asia is neglected. However, pharmaceutical drugs are often used by PWID together or interchangeably with their drug of choice, both orally and by injection. Such use is common when the drugs of choice are in short supply or when a cheaper and easily obtained option is sought.

For example, in the Philippines:

> *Changes in the price of drugs (sniffed/snorted/inhaled) led to an increase in injecting drug use.*
>
> *The price of shabu or methamphetamine soared to P600, while the price of Nubain, the most common injection drug, was only P20 per 0.1 ml (usual injecting dose). Thus, some shabu users shifted to injecting nubain, which is a lot cheaper.*[o]

Unlike in many countries where heroin is the preferred opioid for injecting, India and its neighbouring countries, especially Nepal, Bangladesh and Pakistan, are noting the growing threat of harmful use of pharmaceutical preparations such as buprenorphine, dextropropoxyphene, pentazocine often "cocktailed" with diazepam and nitrazepam, and antihistamines (chlorpheniramine maleate and promethazine) by a considerable proportion of injectors.[p] The illicit and unregulated use of prescription medication has also been reported in many countries of Asia, including some Pacific islands (e.g. Fiji, Papua New Guinea, Samoa and Tonga), though not necessarily by injection.[62]

This lack of attention results in non-inclusion of prevention and treatment of the use of pharmaceutical drugs as a key component in prevention and information services for harm

---

o   Personal communication, Dr M. Salva (WHO Philippines)

p   Kumar S. Injecting of pharmaceutical drugs in the SAARC region: a review. New Delhi, UNODC Regional Centre, 2007. (unpublished)

reduction, and a lack of psychosocial support for users of harmful pharmaceuticals. This omission should be addressed in the next five years.

C.3.4 Addressing emerging drug use and concomitant HIV/AIDS in the Pacific Islands and Territories

The main drugs used in the Pacific Island states are licit drugs, notably alcohol as well as traditional psychoactive substances such as kava. However, the inclusion of the Pacific in this strategy is more than tokenism. In the next five years, it is critical to focus on the emerging patterns of substance use in these islands and assist in the development of culturally appropriate approaches to prevent the spread of drug use and HIV in the region. With the absence of effective national and regional drug data surveillance systems, new patterns of and trends in drug use may emerge and become prevalent before effective responses are initiated.

The Burnet Institute together with the Australian National Council on Drugs (ANDC) are collecting strategic information to inform the development of preventive strategies.[63] These should be monitored and evaluated as an integral part of the regional strategy.

C.3.5 Addressing the lack of attention to drug overdose among out-of-treatment PWID

Although drug overdose is one of the main causes of morbidity and mortality among PWID, research on this matter is scant. The rate of accidental, fatal and non-fatal overdose is unknown. Studies have indicated that mixing of heroin with central nervous system depressants such as benzodiazepines, younger age, purity of the drug, injection drug use, history of imprisonment or detoxification, social marginalization, homelessness and HIV positivity were all associated with non-fatal drug overdose, though evidence of causal association could not be established.[63]

Data from Viet Nam indicate that mortality due to all causes among PWUD in Ho Chi Minh City and Hanoi during a nine-month period in 2001 was 1.9% and 0.9%, respectively. A study in Viet Nam in 2008 found that among 299 PWID in two districts of Bac Ninh province, prevalence of lifetime and recent non-fatal overdose was 43.5% and 83.1%, respectively.[64] The authors of the study note that, given the considerable prevalence of non-fatal overdoses, overdose prevention and management interventions should be considered for inclusion as a standard component of HIV prevention. It can also be assumed that some overdoses may turn out to be fatal.

D. Developing national harm reduction strategies

Key considerations

As already noted, this regional strategy is conceptualized as a framework designed to assist national governments and programmes to develop their own "business plans" and "road maps". In order to achieve the goals and objectives of this strategy, and meet the MDGs, it will be necessary to continue with both regional- and national-level advocacy for expanded harm reduction services to reach universal access. As already noted, although accepted in principle, it is far from being mainstreamed into national responses to prevention and care for PWID. It is necessary for stakeholders to agree on objectives, targets, a workplan, and common indicators by which to assess progress. In considering the way forward, it is important to not only consider whether interventions are ethical, evidence based and respect human rights but also whether they are economically viable, cost-effective and sustainable.

D.1 Are the proposed interventions cost-effective?

In view of the limited availability of financial resources, it is critical for governments to examine the cost-effectiveness of interventions. However, the Independent Commission on AIDS in Asia recommended that governments prioritize programmes that are high impact, whether they are "low cost" or "high cost", and that a focused prevention package among PWID could halve needle-sharing and the percentage of actual injections that PWID share.[32] The Commission further argued that such behaviour changes, if achieved among PWID and other populations at high risk, would result in a significant reduction in cumulative HIV infections, the number of PLHIV, AIDS-related deaths and a decline in HIV prevalence in the region. The Commission estimated that 80% of new HIV infections could be averted through a focused response as recommended.[32]

A significant body of evidence on the cost-effectiveness of harm reduction interventions (NSP, OST, condom programme, with referral to VCT and ART) is available internationally. A global review of the effectiveness of drug dependence treatment in preventing HIV/AIDS among PWID by WHO (2005)[65] concluded that there is clear evidence that MMT reduces HIV risk behaviour. The findings of the global review indicate a cross-study average of 76% reduction in the annual number of injections per PWID and 67% reduction in needle-sharing. Further examples of research findings from studies in countries of Asia are provided in Table 1 Annex 4. These conclusively demonstrate significant reductions in high-risk behaviours among PWID who participate in NSP and OST programmes.

D.2 Can HIV infection be averted through the provision of NSP and OST?

Several countries in Asia have estimated the number of HIV and hepatitis C infections that have been prevented by NSP and MMT. The following are some examples:

- In Bangladesh, it was estimated that NSP might have reduced the incidence of HIV by 90% among PWID.[66]
- In China, it is estimated that the pilot MMT programme prevented HIV among PWID. HIV prevalence among PWID who participated was 0% while among those who did not participate in the MMT programme it was 8.8% in Xinjiang, 4% in Yunnan and 3.1% in Guangxi. The Government of China has reported that in 2008, the national MMT programme averted an estimated 3377 HIV infections.[67]
- In Viet Nam, the estimated number of HIV infections prevented over a four-year period from a range of harm reduction interventions (peer education/outreach, drop-in centres, methadone clinics and methadone provided in existing facilities) was 1286.[q] It was estimated that the annual reduction in injecting per PWID in methadone treatment was 76% and the percentage reduction in sharing of injection paraphernalia was 67%.[r]
- In Australia, between 2000 and 2007, NSP prevented 32 050 HIV cases and 96 667 cases of hepatitis C.[68]

D.3 What is the cost–benefit of averting HIV and hepatitis C?

The assessment of the cost of what is prevented is based on complex mathematical modelling and projections based largely on sets of assumptions and probabilities. Medical, social and economic costs vary from country to country and change over time; however, the savings are impressive. The examples below are illustrative.

---

q   Existing facilities, such as TB, ART or VCT clinics or district health centres could be used to distribute methadone. Cost and administrative efficiencies would be achieved through utilizing existing infrastructure, medical storage, staff, patient management and financial systems.

r   Access Economics/The Nossal Institute for Global Health. Economic appraisal of HIV/AIDS prevention programs in Vietnam. Prepared for the UK Department for International Development. March 2009 (unpublished report)

Analysis of cost–benefits from NSP and OST programmes
In Viet Nam,[69] the lifetime costs of HIV illness were estimated for direct and indirect costs:[s] Direct costs were estimated at US$ 3049 (ART US$ 1895 and hospital treatment US$ 1153). Indirect costs were estimated at US$ 8554 (reduction in employment for caregivers US$ 349 and permanent reduction in employment due to premature death US$ 8205).   The disability-adjusted life-year (DALY) index for PWID in Viet Nam was calculated at 25.8 years (21.7 years due to premature death and 4 years due to disability).   An analysis of cost–benefit for two delivery models for methadone – the methadone clinic, and methadone delivered in health-care facilities – demonstrated that savings for the methadone clinic (from the donor perspective) for four years was US$ 125 565 (294 cases prevented), and for methadone provided as part of an HIV package of interventions in a health centre it was calculated at US$ 142 722.
In Bangladesh (Dhaka), the cost-effectiveness of harm reduction interventions for PWID over a three-year period was assessed. It was estimated that the cost per HIV infection prevented over a three-year period was US$ 110.4 (range: US$ 33.1–182.3).[70]
In Australia, between 2000 and 2007, the cost of NSP was Aus. $ 243 million. However, it is estimated that the net financial saving was Aus $ 1.03 billion. For every dollar invested in NSP, more than four dollars were returned in health-care cost-savings in the short term (10 years). However, if patient costs and productivity gains and losses are included in the analysis, it was estimated that for every one dollar invested in the NSP, $27 is returned in cost savings.[68]
In India the estimated cost of treatment for HCV was US$ 12 000 in 2009.[71]

A different analysis in Thailand[72] estimated that the legacy of weak prevention, if continued, is likely to produce about 1000 new PWID infections in the next decade unless prevention efforts are strengthened substantially.

Existing analysis provides convincing evidence that NSP and OST are not only a humane approach to drug problems but also a convincing and economically prudent approach that mitigates the costs of HIV and hepatitis C treatment. It is salutary to remember that these interventions also prevent transmission from PWID to their partners and children.

A note on expected outcome: The strategy at both the regional and national levels will be closely monitored and evaluated. As each country has its own monitoring and evaluation (M&E) system, it is proposed that basic indicators from the UNGASS reporting system be utilized and that regional guidelines for M&E of harm reduction services in Asia and the Pacific be accorded special attention.

---

s   Economic appraisal of HIV. Final report for DFID (unpublished)

E. Goal and objectives of the strategy for Asia and the Pacific

The goal
Halt and reverse the HIV epidemic among PWID in Asia and the Pacific.

Objective 1

To create an enabling legal and policy environment for implementation of "universal access" and "harm reduction"; increasing support to national governments to adopt critical policy and legal reforms to reconcile public security and a public health approach.

Objective 2

To scale up evidence- and community-based, quality, voluntary HIV prevention, treatment and care services including overdose prevention and management.

Objective 3

To improve the availability and use of quality strategic information to inform evidence-based and cost-effective responses to HIV in the context of injecting drug use.

E.1 Development of a national "business" plan

Guidance on how to develop national plans is provided below. It is proposed that the process should be a step-by-step approach, which initially takes stock of the country situation and what has been done, and identifies gaps in both information and services. Based on this information, planning for the future can begin. At this stage, it is important to consider the barriers to future scaling up of services and ways of overcoming systemic, financial and human resource barriers to expansion of services.

The basic ingredient of the "business plan" for each country should include the following:

- Step I: Analysis of the data on drug use, HIV, hepatitis B and C, and TB
  - Available data: what is known on prevalence and behaviours
  - What are the knowledge gaps
  - What are the emerging issues in the country (e.g. new trends in drug use)

- What is the current level of service coverage
- Step 2: Addressing the barriers to scaling up of harm reduction services
  - Legal and policy barriers
  - Resource barriers (financial/human)
  - Strategic information
  - Advocacy needs
- Step 3: Setting realistic targets for 2010–2015
- Step 4: Developing a costed national plan

An elaboration of the list above of needed actions for the development of a National Business plan is given below.

E.1.1 Step 1: Analysis of data on drug use, HIV, hepatitis B and C, and TB: strategic information

The review should examine both the epidemiological data on drug use and HIV and hepatitis C prevalence, as well as programme coverage and outcome data. The review, which will underpin the development of a national plan, should thus be an analysis of the situation including information gaps, and enable at least a preliminary analysis of what the emerging priorities are. The development of an overarching vision of what the programme should contain in 2010–2015 should emerge from this analysis.

As reliable information on drug use is not easily available, this endeavour remains a challenge and includes uncertainties about who should be counted and how. It is important, therefore, for planners to collect data from multiple sources, e.g. from community groups, networks of PWUD and PLHIV, service providers in medical facilities and NGOs, compulsory centres for drug users, prisons and detention centres. These data would have to be triangulated in order to provide the "best" picture of the country/province situation.

Some guidelines have been developed on the methods of estimation and analysis of drug-use behaviours. Examples of prominent approaches include the rapid assessment and response (RAR) and the RAR-sex analysis (2002).[73,74] In addition, integrated HIV/STI biological and behavioural surveillance surveys (IBBS) have been shown over several years to make an important and useful contribution to informing the national response to HIV. These surveys use reliable methods to track HIV risk behaviours over time as part of an integrated surveillance system, which monitors various aspects of the epidemic. They can be especially useful in providing information on behaviours among subpopulations such as PWUD. In practice, however, these surveys, when employed, do not routinely sample PWUD.

- **Establishing monitoring and evaluation, and measuring outcome and impact**

    Ongoing M&E of all interventions is essential if quality is to be assured. Much of the M&E currently undertaken is guided by the requirements of funding bodies and is focused on ensuring accountability that funds are well spent. It will be necessary to ensure that donors' requirements for data are harmonized with those of the country to avoid the creation of parallel and confusing reporting systems. Furthermore, there is no adequate analysis of treatment costs (for example, comparing the costs of compulsory drug "treatment" with OST programmes). In general, with the exception of selected "good practice" reports, data are lacking on the successes or failures of interventions. It is critical to understand why clients drop out of services (or continue attending) and what happens to them in the medium and long term. In order to achieve this, countries should institute routine and regular follow-up procedures which are built into the national plan.

Each of the priority areas outlined in the UNAIDS Outcome Framework (2009),[26] which are included in the national strategy, represents a distinct goal and requires a combination of specific actions tailored to the country's specific epidemic and building on local capacity. Each of these priority areas requires careful M&E so that the comprehensiveness of the response can be analysed when the strategy is reviewed. A mix of quantitative and qualitative indicators plus composite indices will be used to undertake such ongoing assessments.

The national strategy should include budget provision for the collection and analysis of epidemiological and service data on drug use and HIV, both in the community and in closed settings including prisons and compulsory centres for drug users.

E.1.2 Step 2: Addressing the barriers to scaling up of harm reduction services

Before a country can set realistic targets for harm reduction and universal access, it is necessary to analyse the barriers to scaling up and consider mechanisms for overcoming them in the next five years.

- **Legal and policy barriers**

    Some of the legal and policy barriers to harm reduction have been outlined above and must be addressed to enable services to be scaled up and integrated into national health and welfare systems. A high-level ministerial meeting to discuss these issues has been proposed as a key regional activity to support national initiatives.

    Recommendation for action: Some countries[42,75] in Asia and the Pacific have already undertaken law and policy reviews but those who have not are encouraged to do so and to examine the discord between policing, control of supply, trafficking and use, and the public health objective of reducing the harm from drug use. While these are likely to continue in the foreseeable future, it may nevertheless be possible to impact positively upon them. This could be done, for example, by undertaking targeted advocacy and raising awareness for harm reduction; training for law enforcement and prison personnel, government drug control agencies, and for personnel in compulsory drug "treatment" centres; and supporting multisectoral national harm reduction task forces at which concerned individuals and agencies can meet to discuss issues and exchange information.

Revision of relevant regulations, laws and policies are urgently needed to ensure that harm reduction services can be developed unhindered by legal complications.

- **Human and financial resource barriers**

    Human resource development: The lack of trained personnel is a major barrier to scaling up harm reduction services in the region. Training is required for direct service providers both in the health and the civil society sector, as well as among law enforcement/police and prison personnel whose cooperation is needed to enable the delivery of many crucial services to PWUD. Training is also required for personnel to undertake the collection of strategic information, and formulate and execute research and evaluation.

    A great deal of training materials, operating procedures, guidelines and information packages are available in the region. Some have been prepared internationally by UN agencies such as WHO/UNODC/UNAIDS/UNICEF while others have been prepared by technical agencies such as the Burnet Institute, and by national ministries and civil society service providers. When needed, these should form the basis for the development of any new materials.

    The task of providing training is complex and should be undertaken by different partners with different expertise. These may include national government ministries, universities and colleges, technical agencies, and UN agencies with national counterparts. Technical assistance in the region may be sought from the regional technical support facility (TSF), which provides specialist technical assistance, as well some by NGOs with expertise in the drug and HIV field. Training and awareness-raising for police, law enforcement and prison officials are a priority and may be provided by UNODC, which has a law enforcement mandate and by some bilateral regional programmes that work on harm reduction in the region (e.g. the HAARP programme). All training must be adequately resourced, and quality and professionalism ensured.

Several areas of training are routinely neglected in the region. These include:
- Training for counsellors: this will become a pressing issue when services for ATS users are introduced and scaled up. It is necessary to introduce sustainable long-term counselling courses into appropriate tertiary institutions and to ensure a career progression for counsellors.
- Training for M&E/research/data analysis to be able to undertake regular programme monitoring and conduct follow ups, analyse processes and outcomes, as well as initiate and execute new and original research on drugs and HIV in countries.

To ensure a high standard of harm reduction service provision, attention should be given to the development of a training programme for academic and professional harm reduction staff leading to formal accreditation.

Financial resources: The enormous shortfall in funding for harm reduction to achieve universal access in the region has been calculated in 2009[76] and was estimated at US$ 0.5 billion, NSP and OST accounting for nearly 70% of the overall regional resource need (much of it for China where the problem is most extensive). The cost of scaling up prevention and care activities from the current levels of coverage to the optimum level of coverage by 2015 is estimated to be nearly US$ 2.5 billion. With the exception of a few countries, external funding accounts for the majority of the national AIDS budgets in the region, raising concerns over sustainability of funding over time in view of changing donor priorities and the impact of the global financial crisis.

It is recommended that countries in the region undertake an assessment of the financial requirements in their own country to meet the challenge of universal access. Major donors in the region must be kept abreast of developments and needs in the region and national governments must be persuaded that funding harm reduction services is not only essential but also cost-effective.

Considerable regional and national advocacy will be required to reduce the cost of hepatitis C treatment. However, for harm reduction programmes to be sustainable, it is important to work towards integrating them into existing health and welfare systems, ensuring that services are funded from national budgets.

E.1.3 Step 3: Setting realistic targets for service provision[24]

The two major interventions necessary to prevent and halt the HIV epidemic among and from PWID – NSP and OST – are currently provided at an unacceptably low level of coverage. Although there is no absolute consensus on the optimum targets for essential interventions, nevertheless, the WHO/UNODC/UNAIDS Technical guide[24] provides guidance on target setting for all nine essential interventions and provides recommendations on how to determine the size of the population that requires services.

Using international guidelines on optimal service needs, together with estimates of the target population and information on existing coverage, targets can be set. Calculating the denominator, i.e. the number of people who need services, is necessary. The Guide proposes that separate estimates of subpopulations be considered. It also recommends that while an NSP may target all PWID, OST programmes should target all dependent opioid users including both injectors and non-injectors.[24] It is therefore necessary to estimate the size of these populations separately when measuring the coverage needs for these interventions.

> **Technical guidelines for setting targets for NSP and OST:[24]**
>
> **Needle/syringe programmes (NSP):**
>
> - Counting the number of PWUD regularly reached by NSP, the WHO/ UNODC/UNAIDS Technical guide proposes that the number of individual clients should be counted and not the number of contacts or occasions of service recorded by NSP services.
> - The WHO/UNODC/UNAIDS Technical guide proposes that PWUD who access the service at least once or more per month should be counted.
> - WHO proposes that ≤20% should be seen as low coverage, ≥20 to ≤60% as medium-level coverage and ≥60% as high coverage.
> - Regarding the number of syringes distributed, the WHO/UNODC/UNAIDS Technical guide indicates that low coverage would be ≤100 per year per PWUD, a medium number would be ≥100 to ≤200 and a high number would be ≥200 per year.
>
> **Opioid substitution therapy (OST)**
>
> - The WHO/UNODC/UNIDS Technical guide notes that OST is available in many forms; the most commonly used are methadone and/or buprenorphine. In countries where several substitution medications are used, all of them should be included when measuring these indicators. OST for non-injecting opioid-dependent people should also be included.
> - The number of sites where treatment is available should be noted.
> - Coverage for PWUD – both injectors and non-injectors – can be characterized as: low coverage: <20%, medium coverage: ≥20 to ≤40% and high coverage: ≥40%
> - It is noteworthy that high target levels are based on the levels of coverage achieved in countries with well-established OST programmes.

Guidance on size estimation methods is available in:

- UNAIDS and WHO. Guidelines for Estimating the Size of Populations Most at Risk to HIV. UNAIDS/WHO Working group on Global HIV/AIDS and STI Surveillance. WHO 2010.
- UNODC Global Assessment Programme on Drug Abuse. Estimating prevalence: indirect methods for estimating the size of the drug problem. Vienna, UNODC, 2003.[77]
- Hickman M et al. Estimating the prevalence of problematic drug use: a review of methods and their application. UN Bulletin on Narcotics, 2002, 54:15–32.[78]
- US Department of Health and Human Services, Centers for Disease Control, GAP Surveillance Team.

Most at risk populations sampling strategies and design tool. Atlanta, HSS-CDC, 2000.[79]

Note: All the information in the section above is adapted from the WHO/UNODC/UNAIDS Technical guide (2009).[24]

E.1.4 Step 4: Developing a "costed" national plan (2010–2015)

Based on a coherent vision of how to achieve universal access, which barriers will have to be overcome and how this may be achieved, a national plan, which is a constituent of the regional strategy, can be drafted. This is invariably a multi-agency collaborative enterprise which needs to remain realistic and based on an analysis of data collected during the process described above.

F. Implementing the regional strategy

The table below provides recommendations for regional-level activities, performance indicators and an indicative budget based on the objectives of the regional strategy.

It is not proposed to include recommendations for country-level activities because these should, of course, be determined by national governments on the basis of agreed priorities. The regional strategy document recommends a number of specific steps to be taken by countries when developing their national plans (see Section E.1). Country-level indicators will be developed in tandem with the national strategies and aligned to existing national M&E frameworks.

Please note: Budgets are indicative only.

Regional-level activities									
Strategic objective	Partners	Performance indicators	Indicative budget (US$)	Time frame					
				2010	2011	2012	2013	2014	2015
Mid-term review and evaluation	Representatives of national governments UN agencies, ANPUD, Global Fund and other development partners	Regional-level strategic objectives met	100 000				✓		
Objective 1: To create a legal and policy environment for implementation of universal access and harm reduction: increase support to governments to adopt critical policy and legal reforms to reconcile public security and public health approaches									
High-level ministerial meetings of public security and public health to discuss the role of each in harm reduction: towards a common vision	UNODC, UNAIDS, WHO, Global Fund to fight AIDS, Tuberculosis and Malaria (Global Fund), ASEAN, South Asian Association for Regional Cooperation (SAARC)	High-level meeting to develop country-led roadmaps for joint activities by public security and public health	100 000	✓	✓	✓ Follow up	✓ Follow up		

Regional-level activities									
Strategic objective	Partners	Performance indicators	Indicative budget (US$)	Time frame					
				2010	2011	2012	2013	2014	2015
Agenda item on drugs and HIV in ASEAN and SAARC senior officials' meetings on drugs	UNODC, UNAIDS	Agenda items on HIV and harm reduction. Progress routinely reviewed		✓	✓	✓	✓	✓	✓
Advocacy for national legal and policy reviews: to amend laws and policies inconsistent with HIV strategies and policies in the interest of public health	UNODC, UNAIDS, ANPUD Asian Forum of Parliamentarians on Population and Development (AFPPD)	National drug legislation reviewed and amended in all countries by 2015 and included in revised legal documents		✓	✓	✓	✓		
High-level advocacy for affordable hepatitis C treatment	WHO, UNODC, UNAIDS Global Fund	Substantial price reduction enabling wide access to treatment		✓	✓				
Provision of technical support to national governments to align drug/HIV policies (including in prisons)	UNODC, WHO, UNAIDS	As above		✓	✓	✓	✓		
Advocacy for allocation of national and development funds for harm reduction services that target drug users	Global Fund, UN	Proportionate/adequate funding allocated		✓	✓	✓	✓	✓	✓
Advocacy for lifting the legal obstacles to comprehensive harm reduction (including the procurement of substitution drugs)	UNODC, WHO			✓	✓	✓			

Regional-level activities									
Strategic objective	Partners	Performance indicators	Indicative budget (US$)	Time frame					
				2010	2011	2012	2013	2014	2015
Objective 2: To scale up evidence- and community-based, quality, voluntary HIV prevention, treatment and care services including overdose prevention and management									
Advocacy/technical support for expansion of voluntary community-based drug treatment services to replace compulsory facilities	UNAIDS, UNODC, WHO		80 000	✓	✓				
Provide support to ANPUD to develop national networks of PWUD and other activities	WHO UNODC Global Fund		250 000	✓	✓				
Regional/multicountry training workshops and study visits on planning, implementation, monitoring and evaluation of the HIV prevention, treatment and care package of services	WHO, UNODC		200 000	✓	✓	✓	✓	✓	✓
Preparation, adaptation and translation of key technical materials and guidelines to support countries in the region	WHO, UNAIDS, UNODC		100 000	✓	✓	✓	✓	✓	✓
Support governments to mainstream services for PWUD and PWID (health services strengthening)	WHO, World Bank, Global Fund			✓	✓	✓			

Regional-level activities									
Strategic objective	Partners	Performance indicators	Indicative budget (US$)	Time frame					
				2010	2011	2012	2013	2014	2015
Promote/provide technical support for the development of integrated services for treatment of substance dependence, HIV, hepatitis B and C, TB, STIs and mental health	WHO		200 000	✓	✓	✓			
Advocacy and technical support to governments to develop health services in prisons	UNODC, WHO, UNAIDS		200 000						
Technical support to develop pilot evidence-based drug treatment for PWUD who use ATS and/or inject pharmaceuticals	WHO, UNODC		300 000	✓	✓	✓	✓	✓	✓
Objective 3: To improve the availability and use of quality strategic information to inform evidence-based and cost-effective responses to HIV in the context of injecting drug use									
Development of regionally agreed M&E frameworks to augment UNGASS indicators	WHO, UNODC		150 000	✓	✓	✓			
Preparation, adaptation and translation of key technical material and guidelines to support countries in the region	WHO, UNAIDS, UNODC		100 000	✓	✓	✓	✓	✓	✓

Regional-level activities									
Strategic objective	Partners	Performance indicators	Indicative budget (US$)	Time frame					
				2010	2011	2012	2013	2014	2015
Technical support to governments for setting targets for interventions recommended by WHO/UNODC/UNAIDS24	WHO, UNODC	Realistic targets set. Targets met	150 000	✓	✓	✓	✓	✓	✓
Technical support to advocate and include PWUD/PWID in national HIV sentinel surveillance	WHO	PWUD and PWID routinely included in all HIV surveillance	50 000	✓	✓	✓			
Technical support to develop an M&E system for resource-constrained countries harmonized with existing national systems	WHO UNAIDS	Functioning M&E systems providing good-quality information on all aspects of interventions for PWID	150 000	✓	✓	✓			
Technical support to develop centres of excellence to enable research on drug use and HIV. Training to researchers and data analysts	WHO, development partners, universities/colleges	Research centres established in all countries in Asia and the Pacific	150 000	✓	✓	✓	✓	✓	✓
Technical support to develop sustainable accredited courses for health practitioners and counsellors in drug prevention and treatment	WHO, development partners, universities and colleges	Sustainable courses established in all countries	200 000	✓	✓	✓	✓	✓	✓
Technical support for size estimations of PWID, measurement of intervention coverage	WHO, UNAIDS	Consensus on size of problem and coverage	100 000	✓	✓	✓	✓	✓	✓

Annex 1: Prevalence of drug use in Asia and the Pacific

Table 1: HIV and hepatitis C prevalence among PWID in selected countries of Asia

Country	Estimated number of PWID	Estimated HIV prevalence among PWID	Estimated hepatitis C prevalence among PWID
Afghanistan	6900,[80] 1431 registered[81]	9%[12]	36.6% for hepatitis C and 6.5 for hepatitis B[82]
Bangladesh	20 000–40 000[83]	0.2–2.25%,[10] 7% of PWID in Dhaka[84] 11% in one neighbourhood in Dhaka[t]	25% (>50% PWID in seven cities were positive for HCV)[85] 66.5%[86]
Cambodia	600–10 000[87]	24%[12]	No information
China	1.8–2.9 million Mean: 2 350 000[88]	6.7–13.4%[89]	61.4%[90](HIV+ HCV – 6.5%)[91]
India	96 463–189 729 male 10 055–33 392 female[92]	7.2% (2007)[93] Maharashtra 24.4%, Manipur 17.9%, Tamil Nadu 16.8% Punjab 13.79%, Delhi 10.10%, Orissa 7.3%, Kerala and West Bengal 7.8%, Chandigarh 8.64%	92% (national) 26–93% individual sites[94]
Indonesia	190 460–247 800 Mean: 219 130[80]	52%[8]	60–98%[94]
Lao PDR	Some reported but no data	0.09%[95]	Not known
Malaysia	205 000[80]	60 248 PWID in 200[u] (2/3 of all infections)	Not known
Maldives	3000 PWUD[96]	Not known	Not known
Myanmar	60 000–90 000[80]	34%[12]	Not known
Nepal	38 750 (2006)[97]	35%[12]	85.5% Kathmandu valley[98]
Pakistan	125 000[99]	23% of PWID in urban settings[100] M. Bahauddin – 52% (sample of 300 street-based PWID)[44] Hyderabad – 30.5%[101] Larkana – 28.5%	89%[94]
Papua New Guinea	7500[102]	No information	No information

t   National AIDS/STD Programme (NASP). National HIV serological surveillance. Bangladesh, Directorate General of Health Services (DGHS), 2007 (unpublished).

u   Malaysia Ministry of Health, 2008.

Country	Estimated number of PWID	Estimated HIV prevalence among PWID	Estimated hepatitis C prevalence among PWID
Philippines	9984–20 316[103]	1%[12]	Study of PWID (2002–2008) 91.7% of 1110 tested were positive for HCV and 0.36% (4/1086) coinfection with HIV[104]
Sri Lanka	40 000 PWUD (1.2% are injectors)[105]	No information	No information
Thailand	38 380[106] (2004 data)	48%[12]	90%[94]
Viet Nam	135 305[94]	20%,[12] 42.4%[107]	74.1% in N. Viet Nam study[107]

Summary data from the Pacific[108]

a. **Proportion of youth in US territories reporting injecting drug use:**

Marshall Islands	Females 14.1% (2007)	Males 15.8% (2007)
American Samoa	Females 3.8% (2007)	Males 8.0% (2007)
Guam	Females 2.1% (2007)	Males 5.4% (2007)
Palau	Females 1.0% (2003)	Males 6.8% (2003)

b. **Percentage of HIV infections attributable to PWID in some Pacific Islands**

Melanesia 5.7%

Fiji 0.5%

New Caledonia 10.1%

Micronesia 3.2%

Guam 4.1%

Table 2: Estimates of PWID in prisons who are HIV positive and have hepatitis B or C[v]

Country	Total prison population (including pre-trial detainees)[109]	HIV prevalence in prison	Hepatitis B and C among prisoners (per 100 000)
Afghanistan	9600 (1/07)	11% in males	1899 hepatitis. C, 5244 hepatitis B
Bangladesh	83 000 (19 September 2008)	0.2% in 1999[110]	No data
Cambodia	10 337 (mid 2007)	3.1% in Phnom Penh 1994[110]	No data
China	1 565 771 (31 December 2005) Sentenced prisoners only + 850 000 in administrative detention		0–4%[18]
India	373 271 (31 December 2006)	1.7% in 2000 0.8% among PWID	1–14% female prisoners and 0–7% male prisoners[97] 5000 (1999) hepatitis C
Indonesia	136 017 (10/08)	22%[17] (2002)	No data
Lao PDR	4020 (mid 2004)	1% in Vientiane (1995)[110]	No data
Maldives	1125 sentenced prisoners only (2004)	Not known	No data
Malaysia	50 305 (2007)	6% (1991–2001)[110]	
Myanmar	65 063 (mid 2007)	No prevalence data but 610 HIV positive in 2004	No data
Nepal	6700 (1 January 2008)	Not known	No data
Pakistan	90 000 (2007) 3630 PWUD (2009)[110]	2.7% in Karachi and 6% among females (1993–1998)[110]	Study in one prison in Punjab in 2009, 232/976 were hepatitis C positive and 50 HIV positive (most PWID)[w]
Sri Lanka	25 537 (31 July 2007)	Not known	No data
Philippines	91 530 (2006)	No data	14 000 hepatitis B
Thailand	166 338 (February 2008)	6% (1993–2003)[110]	No data
Viet Nam	98 556 (mid 2006)	0.28% among PWID	28.4%[18]

---

v   Unpublished data from UNODC (Vienna) - where specific references were known these were added.

w   Gordon Mortimore, personal communication, November 2009.

Table 3: Clients in compulsory centres for drug users in selected countries

Country	Number of centres	Number of people in the centres	Date
Bangladesh[x]	6 +	5865[111,y]	2010
Cambodia	11[13] (6 run by military police)[z]	> 2000[aa]	2010
China	717[52]	269 000[52]	2006
Lao PDR	49[ab]	875[ac]	2008
Malaysia	28[52]	7135[52] 5939 new admissions and 6413 repeat admissions (2008)[13]	2007
Myanmar	69[ad]	566[ae]	Jan–June 2009
Thailand	86[af]	16 445[af]	2010
Viet Nam	84[112]	60 000[112]	June 2007

Table 4: Amphetamine-type stimulant (ATS) use in selected countries of Asia

Country	ATS use in general population	% PWID among ATS users	% ATS/HIV/ PWID	Comments/source of information
Bangladesh	No information	No information	No information	Sporadic reports of ATS trafficking and use in major cities in 2007, including reports of high purity crystal methamphetamine. In 2008, 5763 tablets were seized.[13]

---

x   Bangladesh – United Nations Regional Task Force on Injecting Drug Use and HIV/AIDS in Asia and the Pacific. Baseline assessment 2009 (unpublished document)

y   2583 in Centres of the Department of Narcotic Control, 2073 Centres of the Directorate of Prisons and 1209 in Centres supported by Family Health International (FHI)

z   Data from NACD (2007) reveals that clients in the centre comprised 47% who used methamphetamine pills and 34% who used crystalline methamphetamine.

aa   National Drug Control Authority. Meeting with Deputy Prime Minister/Chairman NACD HE Ke Kim Yn, 19 January 2010

ab   UNODC Lao Country Office, personal communication, February 2010

ac   Somsanga centre 800, Champasak centre 20–30, Savanakhet centre 20–30, Oudomxay 20–30

ad   Personal communication, UNODC Myanmar Country Office, 29 January 2010

ae   Personal communication, UNODC Myanmar Country Office, November 2009

af   Presentation by Tanita Nakin on 27 January 2010, Office of the Narcotic Control Board, Thailand

Country	ATS use in general population	% PWID among ATS users	% ATS/HIV/ PWID	Comments/source of information
Cambodia	0.6% (2004) to 20 000 (2005)	12% of street children (2000)[113]	1% of non-injectors 24% of PWID	Methamphetamine use (pill form) is the largest drug problem (reported by 81% of PWUD[113]) Crystal methamphetamine use is increasing. Some inject. Most PWID share needles and syringes.
China	47% of "new" type PWUD (predominantly methamphetamine)[114]	11% (2005)	No information	Use increasing. PWID account for 41% of HIV prevalence
Indonesia	0.3% (2005)	Among those who ever used drugs, use of ATS accounted for 21% (15% crystalline methamphetamine, 9% Ecstasy)[115]	No information	Use increasing. Fourth-largest problem. Typically smoked

In 2006, 9.2% of total admissions for treatment were for methamphetamine dependence.[13] |
| India | 0.02% (2001) 0.03% (2004) National survey | 0% use among PWID (2002) | No information | Some availability reported. Domestic manufacture reported, leading to the possibility of spread of ATS use in young affluent urban population[13] |
| Lao PDR | 0.6% (2008), 90 000 youth 13–21 years estimated to be using ATS.[116] Prevalence is highest in urban and border provinces – an estimated 1.4% in Vientiane Province and 1.1–1.5% in Luang Prabang, Lang Namtha, Bokeo and Houanphanh.[116] | First injected in 200813

30 000–40 000 estimated to be "addicted" to ATS[13] | No information | Pills primary form of drug use; methamphetamine typically smoked |
| Malaysia | 0.6%[117] | 10% of MMT patients are regular users | No information | Fourth most common drug used |
| Myanmar | Not much data. However, arrests related to methamphetamine pills increased from 24% in 2007 to 28% in 2008 (almost as high as for heroin, which is 31%)[13] | No information | No information | Generally smoked – only methamphetamine use has been reported to be increasing for the entire six-year period from 2003 to 2008[13] |

Annex 1

Country	ATS use in general population	% PWID among ATS users	% ATS/HIV/ PWID	Comments/source of information
Philippines	Past year use of methamphetamine in the general population (aged 15–64 years) is between 1.9% and 2.4% (2007 household survey)[13]	But 2007 estimates are 9984–20 316 methamphetamine injectors[13]	<1% (2006) in Cebu (range 0.07–2.17%)	Declining trend in methamphetamine use Typically smoked Treatment admissions have declined from 6195 in 2003 to 2014 in 2008[13]
Thailand	Methamphetamine, Ecstasy or crystal methamphetamine used by 87 755, and 26 758 used in previous 30 days[13]	9% of PWID (2000) 49% of PWID in Bangkok (2004)	2% of PWID	Crystal methamphetamine largest drug problem Generally smoked but also injected, which is common among PWID in Bangkok
Viet Nam	0.2% (2003) crystal methamphetamine use first reported in 2008[13]	Methamphetamine users account for 4% of registered users in 200813,118 not necessarily injectors[13]	No information	Second-largest drug problem, usually oral use Increase in trafficking through Viet Nam

Table adapted from: Reference Group to the United Nations on HIV and injecting drug use. The global epidemiology of methamphetamine injection: a review of the evidence on use and association with HIV and other harms. National Drug and Alcohol Research Centre, University of New South Wales, 2007.[119]

Additional data from the 2009 UNODC report on Patterns and trends of amphetamine-type stimulants and other drugs in East and South-East Asia are referenced separately.[13]

Table 5: HIV risk behaviours among PWID in selected countries of Asia

Country	Percentage of PWID who reported the use of sterile injecting equipment the last time they injected[12]	Percentage of PWID reporting the use of a condom the last time they had sexual intercourse[12]
Afghanistan	…	…
Bangladesh	32	43
Cambodia	66	68–79
China	…	…
India	29–88	44–100
Indonesia	82	34
Lao PDR	…	…
Malaysia	…	…
Maldives	…	…
Myanmar	81	78
Nepal	93	58
Pakistan	77	31
Philippines	48	…
Sri Lanka	…	…
Thailand	…	…
Viet Nam	89	57

Annex 2: Responding to drugs and HIV/AIDS: key international and regional commitments to universal access and harm reduction

I. International commitment to universal access and harm reduction

A number of international and regional commitments and frameworks adopt harm reduction principles for the implementation of HIV and harm reduction activities.

A. United Nations General Assembly Special Session (UNGASS) on HIV and AIDS[21]

The Declaration of Commitment on HIV/AIDS by the United Nations General Assembly 26th Special Session (UNGASS) 27 June 2001 calls inter alia for an expansion of access to sterile injecting equipment and to harm reduction efforts related to drug use (para 52). The UNGASS Guidelines on the Construction of Core Indicators[120] states that:

> *"National governments, through their National AIDS Councils (NACs) or equivalent, are responsible for compiling the national-level indicators with support from UNAIDS and its partners.*

and

> *"Completed forms should be returned to the UNAIDS Secretariat in Geneva. These completed forms should be accompanied by a narrative report highlighting success, as well as constraints and future national plans of action to improve performance, specifically in areas where data indicate weaknesses against national targets intended to monitor the implementation of the Declaration."*

With respect to PWID, the focus is on safe injecting and sexual practices. Thus, the core indicators are focused on percentages of PWID who have adopted behaviours that reduce the transmission of HIV, i.e. who both avoid sharing injecting equipment and use condoms. Specifically, data are requested on whether drugs were injected some time in the past month, whether in the past month PWID avoided sharing injecting equipment, whether they had sexual intercourse in the past month and whether they used condoms. Additionally, countries are expected to collect data on the percentage of PWID who report using sterile injecting equipment and condoms, and are reached with HIV prevention education and information, as well as the percentage of PWID who have been voluntarily tested for HIV.

B. The UNGASS Declaration was followed up by the Resolution of the United Nations General Assembly High-Level Meeting on HIV/AIDS[22] (June 2006), which reaffirmed the commitment of Heads of State and Government representatives of the States and Governments.

> *Pursuing all necessary efforts to scale up nationally driven, sustainable and comprehensive responses to achieve broad multisectoral coverage for prevention, treatment, care and support, with full and active participation of people living with HIV, vulnerable groups, most affected communities, civil society and the private sector, towards achieving the goal of universal access to comprehensive prevention programmes, treatment, care and support by 2010.*

Universal access for PWUD to all HIV and AIDS treatment is articulated in the WHO/UNAIDS[23] Care and treatment for people who inject drugs in Asia and the Pacific: an essential practice guide, which states that

" ART is as effective for people who inject drugs as for other people with HIV/AIDS."

"Given appropriate support, former and current users of injection drugs can adhere to and have equal success on ART."

Universal access must be more than a "wish list" and should be implemented through a concrete process of identifying critical barriers to scaling up, and making plans to address these issues. Universal access encompasses the principles of equality, sustainability, comprehensiveness, accessibility and sustainability. Thus:

- Services should be physically accessible and available including in prisons and other closed settings.
- Services must be affordable.
- Services must be equitable and non-discriminatory with no exclusion criteria, except on medical grounds.
- Treatment should not be rationed: supply should be determined by need and not limited by cost or other considerations.
- Access should not be determined by sociodemographic factors such as age, sex/gender, sexual orientation and sexual behaviour, citizenship, race/ethnicity, asylum-seeking, refugee status, employment status and profession (including sex work).

All interventions should be offered voluntarily in an enabling environment created by supportive legislation, policies and strategies.[24]

C. UNAIDS Programme Coordinating Board

However, in a recent meeting of the UNAIDS governing body, the Programme Coordinating Board (PCB) (2009)[25] noted that major gaps remain in the response to PWUD. NSP and OST still face serious challenges in implementation, particularly where they are not legal or inconsistent with national policing practices. Among the eleven key recommendations were the following:

- *Request the UNAIDS cosponsors and the Secretariat, in particular UNODC, to work with national governments to address the **uneven and relatively low coverage** of services among injecting drug users and to develop comprehensive models of appropriate service delivery for injecting drug users; and (i)*
- *Request… to support national authorities **to align policies, clarify roles and responsibilities of various national entities – including drug control, the penitentiary system, public health and civil society** …(v) and*
- *Recognizing that **existing data on HIV and drug use are far from adequate** in both quality and quantity, requests UNAIDS to support greater investment in data collection required to inform the development of HIV prevention, treatment, care and support initiatives; (viii)*
- *Recognizing that stimulant drug use is a rapidly growing problem, request UNAIDS to strengthen the work on HIV and stimulant drugs.*

The Regional Strategy for Asia and the Pacific will synthesize these key recommendations towards reaching a coherent response to drugs and HIV in the region.

C.1 UNAIDS Outcome Framework 2009–2011[26]

"This outcome framework affirms the UNAIDS Secretariat and cosponsors to leverage respective organizational mandates and resources to work collectively to deliver results." The nine priority areas are interlinked. They include

- Reducing the sexual transmission of HIV,
- Protecting PWUD from becoming infected with HIV,
- Removing punitive laws, policies and practices, stigma and discrimination that block effective responses to AIDS, and
- Ensuring that PLHIV receive treatment.

The framework outlines cross-cutting strategies which call for joint action. These include bringing AIDS planning and action into the national development policy and broader accountability frameworks; optimizing UN support for applications to and from programme implementation of the Global Fund; improving the generation, analysis and use of strategic information country by country, including through the mobilization of novel sources; assessing and realigning the management of technical assistance programmes; developing shared messages for sustained political commitment, leadership development and advocacy; and broadening and strengthening engagement with communities, civil society and networks of PLHIV at all levels of the response.

D. Human Rights Council resolutions (September 2009)

- Resolution A/HRC/12/L.24:[29] Protection of human rights in the context of human immunodeficiency virus
- (HIV) and acquired immunodeficiency syndrome (AIDS). Recalls and reaffirms the commitment to expand "access to essential commodities including … sterile injecting equipment" and "harm reduction efforts related to drug use".

Resolution A/HRC/12/L.23:[28] Access to medicines in the context of the right of everyone to the enjoyment of the highest attainable standard of physical and mental health calls for "ensuring access to all, without discrimination, of medicines, in particular, essential medicines".

E. The United Nations Commission on Narcotic Drugs[ag] Report of the CND[27] (Economic and Social Council)

The ECOSOC met in March 2009 to conclude a two-year review on the global drug control system and progress on the UN General Assembly's declaration which, at its twentieth special session (1998), included "making measurable progress in demand reduction".[121] Consequently, it issued a report in which they

> "Note with great concern the adverse consequences of drug abuse for individuals and society …also note with great concern the alarming rise in the incidence of HIV/AIDS and other bloodborne diseases among injecting drug users, reaffirm our commitment to work towards the goal of **universal access to comprehensive prevention** programmes and treatment, care and related support services, in full compliance with the international drug control conventions and in accordance with national legislation, taking into account all relevant General Assembly resolutions and, when applicable, the WHO, UNODC, UNAIDS Technical guides."

and:

> "Consider developing a comprehensive treatment system offering a wide range of integrated pharmacological (such as detoxification and opioid agonist and antagonist maintenance) and psychosocial (such as counselling, cognitive behavioural therapy and social support) interventions based on scientific evidence and focused on the process of rehabilitation, recovery and social reintegration."

---

ag The Commission on Narcotic Drugs (CND) was established by the UN Economic and Social Council (ECOSOC) in 1946 and is the main drug policy-making body within the United Nations system. It has the power to influence drug control policy by advising other bodies and deciding how various substances will be controlled. It consists of representatives from 53 States.

II. Regional commitment to harm reduction in Asia

A. ASEAN commitments on HIV and AIDS

ASEAN comprises representatives from ten countries in South-East Asia. It provides a regional forum for governments to discuss national and regional matters including the issues presented by HIV/AIDS and drugs. In October 2000, it issued the Bangkok Political Declaration in pursuit of a drug-free ASEAN 2015[122] in which it

> "Affirm[ed] the need for an inter-sectoral plan of action with clear objectives, measurable targets, collectively owned by the international community that will enable us to execute the necessary actions towards the achievement of our common goal of a drug-free ASEAN 2015."

Following on the pursuit of a drug-free ASEAN of 2000, the Commitments on HIV and AIDS (2007–08)[30,31] reflect a willingness in ASEAN countries to focus efforts on providing services to PWUD to prevent HIV infection. This commitment is also reflected in the workplan programme on HIV and AIDS III (2006–2010) in which the need to protect the health of PWID, their partners, families and communities, by facilitating all effective means (including access to clean needles and syringes) to prevent the spread of bloodborne viruses including HIV is acknowledged.

B. Redefining AIDS in Asia: crafting an effective response

However, the report of the Independent Commission on AIDS in Asia (2008),[32] which was established by UNAIDS, notes that although countries should "Facilitate and support the introduction of integrated comprehensive harm-reduction programmes" (p. 35) that

> "… these measures are not always politically popular, but their effectiveness is beyond dispute. If introduced on a large-enough scale, they can contribute significantly to reducing the HIV epidemics in countries where injecting drug use is common". (p. 199)

It notes that:

> "Of the 11 countries in Asia with drug-related HIV epidemics, no country currently offers a comprehensive harm reduction programme that includes both drug substitution and needle (and syringe) exchange services on the required scale. Most of these countries offer one or the other of those services, which is inadequate and less effective."

Annex 2

C. The UNODC Regional Programme Frameworks

East Asia and the Pacific (2009–2012)[33]

The UNODC framework and workplan for East Asia and the Pacific tackles several of the key priorities and objectives of the present regional strategy for Asia and the Pacific. The main objective of UNODC in the Health and Development thematic area in the subprogramme on HIV/AIDS is to address the low coverage, poor information and little mainstreaming of HIV services for PWUD. It proposes to focus on areas where it has a comparative advantage. These are:

- Identification of local champions and the development of local-level partnerships in areas of criminal justice, HIV/AIDS prevention, treatment and care

- Advocacy in a number of areas, including (a) the establishment of high-level committees on correctional settings and HIV/AIDS; (b) the right to health; (c) prison reform (where applicable); (d) drug control legislative/policy review (including alternatives to imprisonment); (e) assessment of criminal justice systems, particularly where compulsory drug treatment systems are in place; and (f) HIV/AIDS prevention, treatment and care

- Research (a) in all correctional settings; (b) into the epidemiological situation; and (c) into the effectiveness and efficiency of different approaches

- Development of partnerships for HIV/AIDS in correctional settings and in criminal justice work, particularly with prison /Corrections Departments, ministries of health and WHO.

South Asia Regional Programme (2008–2011)[34]

The UNODC programme for South Asia includes the key area of HIV/AIDS prevention and care as related to PWID, in prison settings and with respect to trafficking in human beings. The programme acknowledges the insufficient coverage of services for PWID and the need for scaling up to universal access. It indicates that UNODC's priority for the programme period is to support national efforts in South Asia (especially in Bangladesh, India and Nepal).

A further major objective of the regional programme is harmonizing the public health and the law enforcement perspective on harm reduction. To achieve this, the UNODC Regional Office for South Asia (ROSA) will encourage a policy dialogue between the two sectors and endeavour to move stakeholders towards a position where care can be provided in an evidence-based manner and in consonance with what the law will allow.

UNODC ROSA will also address drug use and HIV in prison settings and will seek to expand services.

Annex 3: Responding to injecting drug use in selected countries of Asia

Table 1: Summary: the state of the response to PWID to prevent HIV and viral hepatitis: NSP

Country	Number of NSP sites	Number of NSP sites per 1000 PWID[12]	Proportion of PWID accessing NSP in a year (%)[123]	Number of PWID accessing NSP in a year[123]	Number N&S per PWID per year[12]
Afghanistan	16 sites in 4 cities (Kabul, Mazar-e-Sharif, Herat and Jalalabad[ah])	0.9		Not known	133 952 NES in 2009[124]
Bangladesh	93 sites[125]	2.3	93	23 684–32 766	101.8
Cambodia	Two NGOs in Phnom Penh provide services[126]	1.0	Not known	Not known	58.8
China	901 sites[127]	Not available	2	>38 000	1 173 764 needles distributed in 200867
India	222 targeted interventions sites in 14 states[92]	1.1	78	137 000	28.6
Indonesia	182 sites[128]	2.7	23	49 000	6.8
Lao PDR	Not available	0	Not known	0	Not available
Malaysia	23 sites[129]	1.0	2	5571	15.9
Maldives	Not available	0	Not known	0	Not available
Myanmar	36 sites[130]	0.2	39	29 411	46.8
Nepal	48 drop-in centres (UNGASS 2010)	1.3	46	13 504	24.4
Pakistan	Nine sites[ai]	0.1	11	15 000	22.2
Papua New Guinea	None	-	Not known	Not known	-
Philippines	Three sites[12]	0.1	5	800	2.5

ah   Gordon Mortimore, personal communication, November 2009

ai   Nai Zindaqi, personal communication, November 2008

Country	Number of NSP sites	Number of NSP sites per 1000 PWID[12]	Proportion of PWID accessing NSP in a year (%)[123]	Number of PWID accessing NSP in a year[123]	Number N&S per PWID per year[12]
Sri Lanka	None	0.0	0	0	
Thailand	Nine sites[aj]	---	<1	413	---
Viet Nam	One or more sites in 382 districts)[131]	10.5	95	140 [254]	181.1

Table 2: Summary: the state of the response to PWID to prevent HIV and viral hepatitis: OST and ART

Country	Number of OST sites	Number of OST recipients per 100 PWID[123]	Number of PWID receiving OST[ak]	Number of PWID receiving ART[123]	Ratio of PWID receiving ART: 100 PWID living with HIV[123]
Afghanistan	One site (Medecins du Monde)[132]	Not known	Not available	Not known	Not known
Bangladesh	MMT pilot being planned	0	0	5	1 (1–3)
Cambodia	One pilot MMT site to open in 2010[al]	0	0	0	0
China	By October 2009, 652 MMT clinics in 25 provinces[67]	3 (4–6)	By October 2009, 231 596 (cumulative patients) 109 523 (currently on treatment)[67]	9300	3 (2–6)
India	47 sites providing buprenorphine[92] No MMT	3 (3–5)	4600 on buprenorphine[92]	Not known	Not known
Indonesia	49 sites[am]	1	2300 on MMT, 500 on buprenorphine[an]	5406	6 (4–9)
Lao PDR	A pilot with tincture of opium substitution	0	0	Not known	Not known

aj   Personal communication from TTAG (March 2010) Mitsampan HRC/Bangkok (TTAG), Chiang Mai/TDN, Ozone/Chiang Rai, Ozone/Bangkok, Ozone/southern Thailand (at least one), Raks Thai/Samut Prakhan, Raks Thai/Bangkok (2), Alden House/Bangkok

ak   Because of lax regulations of medicines and sales, and of physicians' prescribing practices and lax reporting requirements, it is difficult to accurately record the number of opiate users who are provided with buprenorphine by private physicians.

al   Graham Shaw, WHO Cambodia, personal communication, May 2010

am   Source: Ministry of Health, Indonesia

an   Indonesian Ministry of Health, personal communication, January 2010

Country	Number of OST sites	Number of OST recipients per 100 PWID[123]	Number of PWID receiving OST[ak]	Number of PWID receiving ART[123]	Ratio of PWID receiving ART: 100 PWID living with HIV[123]
Malaysia	151 sites[129]	2 (2–3)	Registered patients: 21 000; 6538 (Jan–Sept 2009)[129]	Not known	Not known
Maldives	One site[133]	Not known	<150 clients	Not known	Not known
Myanmar	Seven sites[134]	1	742[135]	Not known	Not known
Nepal	One site[134]	1 (<1–2)	104 MMT patients +30 buprenorphine clients	Not known	Not known
Pakistan	Not available	0	0	113	<1
Papua New Guinea	-	NK	-	Not known	Not known
Philippine	Not available	0	0	Not known	Not known
Sri Lanka	Not available	0	0	Not known	Not known
Thailand	134 sites[134]	3 (2–4)	4000–5000 MMT + 150 clients on buprenorphine[134]	1435	2(1–4)
Viet Nam	Seven sites	1	1475[131]	1760	4 (1–86)

Table 3: Knowledge about HIV and prevention activities

Country	Percentage of PWID who both correctly identify ways of preventing HIV transmission and who reject major misconceptions[ao]	Percentage of PWID reached with HIV prevention programmes in the past 12 months[12]	Percentage of PWID who received HIV testing in the past 12 months and know the result[ao]
Afghanistan	…	…	6
Bangladesh	20	2	3
Cambodia	…	56	…
China	…	…	41
India	14–77	10–83	3–70
Indonesia	58	45	36
Lao PDR	…	…	…
Malaysia	98	…	100
Maldives	…	0	…
Myanmar	…	53	…
Nepal	66	31	8.0
Pakistan	<25 years old: 17 >25 years old: 21	51	<25 years old: 5 > 25 years old: 4
Philippines	…	14	…
Sri Lanka		…	…

ao   Data from Country universal access progress reports, 2008

Country	Percentage of PWID who both correctly identify ways of preventing HIV transmission and who reject major misconceptions[ao]	Percentage of PWID reached with HIV prevention programmes in the past 12 months[12]	Percentage of PWID who received HIV testing in the past 12 months and know the result[ao]
Thailand	49	…	…
Viet Nam	38	43	11

The indicator describing the percentage of PWID reached by prevention programmes in the previous 12 months includes the following:

- Do you know where you can go if you wish to receive an HIV test?
- In the previous 12 months have you been given condoms (e.g. through an outreach service, drop-in centre, or sexual health clinic)?
- In the previous 12 months have you been given sterile needles and syringes (e.g. by an outreach worker, peer educator or from a needle and syringe programme)?

Annex 4: Are NSP and OST effective in reducing high-risk behaviours?

Table 1: Summary of findings from studies of NSP and OST in Asia

Reduction in high-risk behaviours
a. Needle and syringe programmes
An evaluation of the pilot NSP in Malaysia found a reduction in the percentage of PWID passing their injecting equipment to others (from 56% at baseline to 43% at follow up) and a reduction in being injected by a "street or port doctor" (from 42% at baseline to 33% at follow up).[136]
In Bangladesh, an evaluation of the NSP found a significant decline in reported levels of needle- or syringe-sharing, from 62% in 1997 to 18% in 2001.[66]
In China, 14.7% of NSP clients reported needle-sharing compared with 43.7% among those who did not participate in the NSP.[6]
In China, an evaluation of a needle social marketing strategy to control HIV among PWID found a significant reduction in needle-sharing behaviours: from 68% at baseline to 35.3% in the intervention community.[6]
In Viet Nam Lan Son Province, peer-based interventions (IEC+NSP) found a reduction in needle-sharing from 47% at baseline to 22% at 12 months.[137]
b. Opioid substitution therapy programmes
In China, an evaluation of the effectiveness of the first eight MMT clinics found a significant reduction in injection drug use reported by MMT patients (from 69.1% to 8.8%).[138]
In Malaysia, the pilot MMT programme showed a reduction in continued opiate use among MMT patients from 45% at baseline to 10.7% at 6 months.[139]

Annex 5: Organizations in Asia of people who use drugs

A. ANPUD – the Asian Network of People who Use Drugs

At the first Asian Consultation on prevention of HIV infection related to drug use, "Response beyond Borders,"[140] the International Network of People who Use Drugs Asia and the Pacific issued a Declaration known as the Goa Declaration (January 2008) reaffirming the principle that "People using drugs are the solution not the problem." It outlined the objectives of civil society to work towards a collaborative and cooperative future strategy and for a harmonized and integrated response from national governments and donor agencies. It also stressed the importance of a unified civil society across the region which would work to strengthen CBOs and responses.

The Declaration calls on governments, various agencies, bilateral and multilateral organizations, CSOs and the general public to provide support in:

> *"Empowering our communities to advocate and protect our rights and to facilitate meaningful participation in decision-making on issues affecting us;*

and for

> *"Supporting, strengthening and encouraging the development of organizations for people who use drugs in communities/countries where they do not exist".*

and most importantly,

> *"Through collective action, we will challenge existing oppressive drug laws, policies and programmes and work with governments and our constituents to formulate evidence-based drug policies that respect human rights and dignity of people who use drugs."*

The meeting was also attended by parliamentarians in the region who issued a Statement of Commitment acknowledging the roles that parliamentarians can play in the development of policies and legislation that support HIV prevention through decriminalizing drug use and providing care and treatment facilities.

The Declaration was followed up by the official establishment of the Asian Network of People who Use Drugs (ANPUD) in October 2009. Pursuant to the profound need "to establish a network of people who use drugs arises from the fact that no group of oppressed people ever attained liberation without the empowerment and involvement of those directly affected". ANPUD's guiding philosophy is based on the principle of meaningful involvement of people who use drugs (MIPUD). It reflects the voices and needs of people who use drugs in Asia and covers South, South-East and East Asia.

ANPUD's goal is that PWUD in Asia should enjoy equal human rights and opportunities for a better quality of life.

ANPUD's objectives are

- Advocate for policy harmonization, decriminalization, reduced stigmatization and discrimination, and access to diverse, locally driven harm reduction approaches.
- Advocate for access to voluntary and ethical drug treatment in the Asia region.
- Advocate for access to hepatitis C treatment for PWUD in the Asia region.
- Collaborate with various like-minded groups, organizations and agencies to promote the effective and meaningful participation of PWUD in the regional and global response to HIV and drug use.
- Promote a platform and common voice for Asian PWUD, through providing representation and coordination on issues at various forums where PWUD should be represented.
- Support the establishment of national-level drug user networks to ensure representation of PWUD at the grass-roots level. Provide expertise and resources.
- ANPUD's objectives and plans reflect the principles already accepted by UNAIDS. ANPUD has thus been set up by PWUD to advocate for their rights and give voice to their networks across Asia. ANPUD has over 150 members throughout the Asian region who are collaborating to influence decisions that affect their lives.

B. The Asian Consortium on Drug use, HIV, AIDS and Poverty (ACDHAP)

ACDHAP organized the Response Beyond Borders (RBB) consultations and regional meetings. The consultations are a unique initiative that have profiled and captured the experiences of PWUD in Asia. RBB is an entirely civil society-driven initiative that brings together all major stakeholders to examine the legal and policy environment for HIV prevention among PWUD, and access to appropriate evidence-informed interventions.

RBB has convened parliamentarians, UN agencies, legal experts, donors, governments, civil society, PWUD and community organizations on a common platform to inform, assess, discuss and plan Asian responses to Asian issues. In January 2010 in Bangkok, the Parliamentarians Forum on Harm Reduction was born. RBB is a novel regional initiative that should be nurtured and supported.

References

1. International Harm Reduction Association. *What is harm reduction?* Accessed on 28 April 2010 at http://www.ihra.net/Whatisharmreduction.

2. Millennium Development Goals. *UN Millennium summit*, September 2000. Accessed on 28 April 2010 at http://www.un.org/millennium/declaration/ares552e.pdf

3. UNAIDS/WHO. *AIDS epidemic update*. Geneva, WHO, 2009.

4. UNAIDS. *World AIDS Day report*. AIDS Outlook /09. Geneva, UNAIDS, 2008.

5. UNODC. *World drug report*. Vienna, UNODC, 2009:58.

6. Wu Z, Yin W. Scaling-up of methadone maintenance treatment (MMT) in China. In: *Proceedings of a Satellite Session on HIV prevention interventions for injecting drug users: lessons learned from Asia*. Organized by the United Nations Regional Task Force on Injecting Drug Use and HIV/AIDS for Asia and the Pacific. 19th International Harm Reduction Conference, Barcelona, 11–15 May 2008.

7. UNAIDS. *UNGASS Country progress report China*. Geneva, UNAIDS, 2008. Accessed on 28 April 2010 at http://www.unaids.org/en/CountryResponses/Countries/China.asp.

8. National AIDS Commission (NAC), Republic of Indonesia. *Country report on the follow-up to the Declaration of Commitment on HIV/AIDS.(UNGASS). Reporting period 2006–2007*. Jakarta, NAC, 2008.

9. Kamarulzaman A. *Rolling out the national harm reduction programme in Malaysia*. In: 9th International Congress on AIDS in Asia and the Pacific. Bali, Indonesia, 2009.

10. Ministry of Health and Family Welfare, Bangladesh. *UNGASS country progress report. Reporting period: January 2006–December 2007*. Dhaka, National AIDS/STD Programme (NASP), 2008.

11. Commission on AIDS in the Pacific. *Turning the tide: an open strategy for a response to AIDS in the Pacific*. Report of the Commission on AIDS in the Pacific, Presented to Ban Ki-Moon, UN Secretary General, New York, 2 December 2009. Bangkok, Commission on AIDS in the Pacific, 2009. Accessed on 01 June 2010 at http://data.unaids.org/pub/Report/2009/20091202_pacificcommission_en.pdf.

12. WHO/UNAIDS/UNICEF. *Towards universal access: scaling up priority HIV/AIDS interventions in the health sector. Progress report 2009*. Geneva, WHO, 2009. Accessed on 28 April 2010 at http://www.who.int/hiv/pub/2009progressreport/en/.

13. UNODC Global SMART Programme. *Patterns and trends of amphetamine-type stimulants and other drugs in East and South-East Asia (and neighbouring regions)*. Vienna, UNODC Global SMART Programme, 2009. Accessed on 22 April 2010 at: http://www.unodc.org/

documents/eastasiaandpacific//2009/11/ats-report/2009_Patterns_and_Trends.pdf

14 Bewley-Taylor D, Hallam C, Allen R; The Beckley Foundation Drug Policy Programme. *The incarceration of drug offenders – an overview. Report* 16. London, King's College, International Centre for Prison Studies, March 2009.

15 Wan Mahmood WMN (Deputy Director General Malaysian Prisons Department). Harm reduction: initiating methadone maintenance therapy in prisons in Malaysia. In: Proceedings of a Satellite Session on HIV prevention interventions for injecting drug users: lessons learnt from Asia. Organized by the UN Regional Task Force on Injecting Drug Use and HIV/AIDS for Asia and the Pacific. 19th International Harm Reduction Conference, 11–15 May, Barcelona, Spain, 2008.

16 WHO, UNODC, UNAIDS. Evidence for Action: interventions to address HIV in prisons: needle and syringe programmes and decontamination strategies. Geneva, WHO, 2007.

17 Oppenheimer E, Gunawan S. A review of vulnerable populations to HIV and AIDS in Indonesia. Jakarta, Indonesia, UNAIDS and National AIDS Commission, 2006.

18 Cook C, Kanaef N. Global state of harm reduction: regional overview: Asia. London, International Harm Reduction Association (IRHA), 2009. Accessed on 02 June 2010 at http://www.ihra.net/Asia.

19 Thomson N et al. Correlates of incarceration among young methamphetamine users in Chiang Mai, Thailand. American Journal of Public Health, 2008, 99:1232–1238.

20 Martin G et al. Does drug rehabilitation in closed settings work in Viet Nam? Presentation at the IHRA Conference 2009, Session on Compulsory drug dependence treatment centres: costs, rights and evidence. Bangkok, Thailand, 2009.

21 United Nations General Assembly 26th Special Session. Declaration of Commitment on HIV/AIDS. Available from http://www.un.org/ga/aids/docs/aress262.pdf (accessed on 01 June 2010).

22 2006 UN High-Level Meeting on AIDS (31 May to 2 June 2006). Accessed on 27 April 2010 at http://www.un.org/ga/aidsmeeting2006/.

23 WHO WPRO/UNAIDS. Care and treatment for people who inject drugs in Asia and the Pacific: an essential practice guide. Manila, the Philippines, WHO WPRO, 2008. Accessed on 28 April 2010 at http://www.wpro.who.int/publications/PUB_9789290613206.htm

24 WHO, UNODC, UNAIDS. Technical guide for target setting for HIV prevention, treatment and care for injecting drug users. Geneva, WHO, 2009. Accessed on 27 April 2010 at http://www.unodc.org/documents/hiv-aids/idu_target_setting_guide.pdf

25 UNAIDS. 24th Programme Coordinating Board (PCB). Geneva, UNAIDS, 2009. Accessed on 27 April 2010 at http://www.unaids.org/en/KnowledgeCentre/Resources/PhotoGal/22062009_PCB_Geneva.asp.

26 UNAIDS. Joint action for results: UNAIDS outcome framework 2009–2011. Geneva, UNAIDS, 2009. Accessed on 27 April 2010 at http://www.unaids.org/en/KnowledgeCentre/Resources/FeatureStories/archive/2009/20090421_Joint_Action.asp.

27 United Nations Economic and Social Council: Commission on Narcotic Drugs. Report on the 52nd session (14 March 2008 and 11–20 March 2009). New York, Official Records 2009, Suppl. No 8 (E/2009/28). Accessed on 27 April 2010 at http://daccess-dds-ny.

un.org/doc/UNDOC/GEN/V09/825/56/PDF/V0982556.pdf?OpenElement.

28. UN General Assembly Human Rights Council. Resolution: A/HRC/12/L.23. Accessed on 27 April 2010 at http://www.idpc.net/sites/default/files/library/Access%20to%20medicines%2012%20HRC.pdf

29. UN General Assembly Human Rights Council. Resolution: A/HRC/12/L.24. Accessed on 27 April 2010 at http://daccess-dds-ny.un.org/doc/RESOLUTION/GEN/G09/174/42/PDF/G0917442.pdf?OpenElement

30. ASEAN. ASEAN commitments on HIV and AIDS. Cebu, Philippines, January 2007. Accessed on 01 June 2010 at http://www.aseansec.org/19322.htm.

31. ASEAN. Vientiane Statement of Commitment on the greater involvement and empowerment of people living with HIV/AIDS. Vientiane, Lao PDR, May 2008. Accessed on 01 June 2010 at http://www.aseansec.org/21863.pdf

32. The Commission on AIDS in Asia. Redefining AIDS in Asia: crafting an effective response. New Delhi, Oxford University Press, 2008. Accessed on 27 April 2010 at http://data.unaids.org/pub/Report/2008/20080326_report_commission_aids_en.pdf.

33. UNODC. Regional Programme Framework for East Asia and the Pacific 2009–2012. Vienna, UNODC Regional Centre for East Asia and the Pacific, 2009. Accessed on 27 April 2010 at http://www.unodc.org/documents/eastasiaandpacific//rceap-response/miniRPF_11_20_Oct_2009LowSol1.pdf.

34. UNODC. Regional Programme for South Asia 2008–2011. Vienna, UNODC Regional Office for South Asia. Accessed on 27 April 2010 at http://www.unodc.org/pdf/india/Regional_Programme_(Aug_2008)_02.pdf.

35. ASEAN. Operational Workplan of the third ASEAN work programme on HIV/AIDS 2006–2010 (AWP III). Accessed on 27 April 2010 at http://www.hivmobilitysea.org/e-library/documents/OperationalWorkPlan-ASEAN.pdf.

36. National Committee for HIV and AIDS Prevention and Alleviation. The national plan for strategic and integrated HIV and AIDS prevention and alleviation 2007–2011: key contents. Bangkok, Thailand, Department of Disease Control, Ministry of Public Health/ United Nations Development Programme, Nov. 2007. Accessed on 01 June 2010 at http://www.whothailand.org/LinkFiles/Areas_of_Work_NAP.pdf

37. UNODC. Prison settings. Accessed on 28 April 2010 at http://www.unodc.org/unodc/en/hiv-aids/prison-settings.html

38. Republic of Indonesia Ministry of Justice. The Indonesian national strategy for HIV/AIDS prevention, care and support for prisoners. Jakarta, Ministry of Justice, 2005.

39. UNHCR/WHO/UNAIDS. Policy statement on HIV testing and counselling in health facilities for refugees, internally displaced persons and other persons of concern to UNHCR. Geneva, UNHCR Public Health and HIV Section, 2009.

40. UNAIDS/UNHCR. HIV and refugees: policy brief. Geneva, UNAIDS, 2007. Accessed on 28 April 2010 at http://data.unaids.org/pub/briefingnote/2007/policy_brief_refugees.pdf

41. Lawyer's Collective HIV/AIDS Unit. A preview of law and policy in South and South East Asia, Drugs, treatment and harm reduction. Background Paper for Response Beyond Borders, the 1st Asian Consultation on Prevention of HIV related Drug Use. Goa, India,

28–31 January, 2008.

42 HIV/AIDS Asia Regional Program (HAARP). Law and policy review. July 2009. Accessed on 27 April 2010 at http://www.haarp-online.org/resources/document/HAARP%20Law%20and%20Policy%202009%20(pdf)(456kb).pdf

43 Decisions taken by UN entities in 2009 concerning injecting drug use and HIV. Available at: http://www.unodc.org/unodc/search.html?q=Decisions+taken+by+UN+entities+in+2009+concerning+injecting+drug+use+and+HIV

44 Nai Zindagi. Rapid situation assessments of HIV prevalence and risk factors among people injecting drugs in four cities in the Punjab (Mandi Bahauddin, Rawalpindi, Gujrawala, Sheikhupura). Published with the assistance of the Punjab AIDS Control Programme, Department of Health, Government of Punjab, Pakistan, 2009.

45 Kumar SM et al. A rapid situation and response assessment of the female regular sex partners of male drug users in South Asia: Factors associated with condom use during the last sexual intercourse. International Journal of Drug Policy, 2008, 19:148–158.

46 Nai Zindagi. The hidden truth – findings of a study of HIV vulnerability, risk factors and prevalence among men injecting drugs and their wives. Published with the assistance of Punjab AIDS Control Programme, Department of Health, Government of Punjab, Pakistan and the Global coalition on Women and AIDS, Geneva, Switzerland, 2008.

47 Panda S et al. Transmission of HIV from injecting drug users to their wives in India. International Journal of STD & AIDS, 2000, 11:468–473.

48 Fazil Z. Rapid situation and response assessment (RSRA) of drug-related HIV in Pakistan, 2008. Project RAS/H13 – Prevention of transmission of HIV among drug users in SAARC countries, supported by AusAID. UNODC Country Office Pakistan, 2009.

49 Yin W, Wu Z. China: government model for taking harm reduction to scale. National Centre for AIDS/STD Control and Prevention, and Chinese Centre for Disease Control and Prevention. Presentation at the 9th ICAAP meeting, Bali, Indonesia, August 2009.

50 APN+. Access to HIV-related health services in positive women, men who have sex with men (MSM), transgender (TG) and injecting drug users (IDU): research findings highlights. Bangkok, Thailand, APN+, August 2009.

51 Human Rights Watch. "Skin on the cable": the illegal arrest, arbitrary detention and torture of people who use drugs in Cambodia. January 2010. Accessed on 28 April 2010 at http://www.hrw.org/en/reports/2010/01/25/skin-cable.

52 World Health Organization Regional Office for the Western Pacific (WHO WPRO). Assessment of compulsory treatment of people who use drugs in Cambodia, China, Malaysia and Viet Nam: an application of selected human rights principles. Manila, the Philippines, WHO WPRO, 2009.

53 UNODC/WHO. Principles of drug dependence treatment: discussion paper. Geneva, UNODC, 2008.

54 Wodak W. Hepatitis C: waiting for the Grim Reaper. Medical Journal of Australia, 1997, 166:284.

55 World Health Organization. Hepatitis C – global prevalence (update). Weekly Epidemiological Record, 1999, 74:425–427.

56 World Health Organization. HIV/AIDS in the South-East Asia Region. New Delhi, WHO, 2007.

57 Avihingsanon A. Coinfection in Thailand. Abstract from NIH/ US–Japan Joint AIDS and Hepatitis meeting, Portland, Oregon USA, October 2009.

58 Singh YS, Chingsubam B. PLHIV among IDUs – dying not with HIV but with HCV in the State of Manipur. Study conducted by the Social Awareness Service Organization (SASO) in Manipur, in collaboration with Fulford, a drug manufacturing company and reported at the International Congress on AIDS in Asia and the Pacific (ICAAP) meeting, Bali, 2009.

59 Tedaldi E et al; The SMART study group and INSIGHT. Opportunistic disease and mortality in patients co-infected with hepatitis C virus (HCV) and/or hepatitis B virus (HBV) in the SMART (Strategic Management of Antiretroviral Therapy) study. Clinical Infectious Diseases, 2008, 47:1476–1478.

60 UNODC. 2007 World drug report. Vienna, UNODC, 2007. Accessed on 28 April 2010 at http://www.unodc.org/unodc/en/data-and-analysis/WDR-2007.html.

61 Centers for Disease Control and Prevention (CDC), Department of Health and Human Services. Methamphetamines use and the risk for HIV /AIDS: Fact Sheet. Atlanta, CDC, January 2007. Accessed on 20 May 2010 at: www.cdc.gov/hiv/resources/factsheets/meth.htm.

62 Devaney M, Reid G, Baldwin S. Situational analysis of illicit drug issues and responses in the Asia–Pacific Region. Canberra, Australian National Council on Drugs, 2006.

63 Regional analysis of drug and alcohol issues and responses in the Pacific. Melbourne, Australia, Burnet Institute, 2009. (Draft report 2008-0).

64 Bergenstrom A et al. A cross-sectional study on the prevalence of non-fatal drug overdose and associated risk characteristics among out-of-treatment injecting drug users in North Vietnam. Substance Use and Misuse, 2008, 43:73–84.

65 WHO. Evidence for action technical paper and policy brief. Effectiveness of drug dependence treatment in preventing HIV among injecting drug users. Geneva, WHO, 2005.

66 Foss AM et al. Could the CARE-SHAKTI intervention for injecting drug users be maintaining the low HIV prevalence in Dhaka, Bangladesh? Addiction, 2007, 102:114–125.

67 Yin W. Scaling-up harm reduction programmes in China. Presented at the meeting on the Development of the regional strategy for harm reduction in Asia and the Pacific 2010–2015 – Confronting HIV among people who inject drugs. Kuala Lumpur, Malaysia, 7–9 December 2009.

68 Australian Government, Department of Health and Ageing, National Centre in HIV Epidemiology and Clinical Research/UNSW. Return on investment 2: evaluating the cost-effectiveness of needle and syringe programs in Australia. 2009. Accessed on 02 June 2010 at http://www.health.gov.au/internet/main/publishing.nsf/Content/C562D0E860733E9FCA257648000215C5/$File/retcov.pdf.

69 Keating C et al.; Access Economics, DFID and The Nossal Institute, Melbourne. Testing the cost-effectiveness of various harm reduction models in Viet Nam. Presentation made

at the International Harm Reduction Conference Bangkok, Thailand, 2009. Accessed on 28 April 2010 at http://www.ihra.net/Assets/1602/1/AbstractsBook_HR2009.pdf.

70. Guinness L et al. The cost-effectiveness of consistent and early intervention of harm reduction for injecting drug users in Bangladesh. Addiction, 2009, 105:319–328.

71. Sohn A. Hepatitis B and C in the Asia–Pacific. Data from the TREAT Asia HIV Observational Database (Quoting from http//www.citizen-news.org/2009/04/major-setback-for-scaling-up-hepatitis.html). Presentation made at the Kuala Lumpur consultation, December 2009.

72. Family Health International (FHI) and Bureau of AIDS, TB and STIs. Asian Epidemic Model (AEM) – projections for HIV/AIDS in Thailand 2005–2025. Bangkok, Thailand, Department of Disease Control, Ministry of Public Health, 2008.

73. WHO.Technical guide to rapid assessment and response (TG-RAR). Geneva, WHO, 2002. Available at: http://www.who.int/hiv/pub/prev_care/tgrar/en/

74. WHO. Sex-RAR guide: the rapid assessment and response guide on psychotropic substances and sexual risk behaviours. Geneva, WHO, 2002. Available at: http://www.who.int/hiv/topics/vct/sw_toolkit/121substancesexrar.pdf

75. Grover A, Tandon T; Lawyer's Collective HIV/AIDS Unit, India. Legal framework in the region: findings from a legal and policy review of IDU harm reduction in SAARC. Presented at the Inter-country Consultation on preventing HIV among IDUs: from evidence to action. Kolkata, India, 10–13 April 2007.

76. Bergenstrom A et al. How much will it cost? Estimation of resource needs and availability for HIV prevention, treatment and care for people who inject drugs in Asia. International Journal of Drug Policy, 2010, 21:107–109.

77. UNODC, Taylor C, Hickman M (editors). Global Assessment Programme on Drug Abuse (GAP) toolkit module 2. Estimating prevalence: indirect methods for estimating the size of the drug problem. Vienna/New York, UNODC/United Nations, 2003.

78. Hickman M et al. Estimating the prevalence of problematic drug use: a review of methods and their application. UN Bulletin on Narcotics, 2002, 54:15–32.

79. US Department of Health and Human Services, Centers for Disease Control, GAP Surveillance Team. Most at risk populations sampling strategies and design tool. Atlanta, HSS-CDC, 2000.

80. Mathers BM et al. Global epidemiology of injecting drug use and HIV among people who inject drugs: a systematic review. The Lancet, 2008, 372(9651):1733–1745.

81. Islamic Republic of Afghanistan, Ministry of Health. National AIDS Control Program consolidated data. Kabul, Ministry of Health, 2009.

82. Todd CS et al. HIV, hepatitis C, and hepatitis B infections and associated risk behavior in injection drug users, Kabul, Afghanistan. Emerging Infectious Diseases, 2007, 13:1327–1331.

83. Reddy A., Hoque MM, Kelly R. HIV transmission in Bangladesh: an analysis of IDU programme coverage. International Journal of Drug Policy, 2008, 19 (suppl 1):S37–S46.

84. Azim T et al. Prevalence of infections, HIV risk behaviors and factors associated with HIV infection among male injecting drug users attending a needle/syringe exchange program

in Dhaka, Bangladesh. Substance Use and Misuse. 2008, 43:2124–2144.

85. Rahman M et al. Co-infection of HIV with hepatitis B and hepatitis C in injecting drug users in Dhaka, Bangladesh. US–Japan Joint AIDS Hepatitis Meeting Abstracts, Oregon, September 2009.

86. Azim T et al. Injecting drug users in Bangladesh: prevalence of syphilis, hepatitis, HIV and HIV subtypes. AIDS, 2002, 16:121–123.

87. National Authority for Combating Drugs. Cambodia National Strategic Plan. Illicit drug use and related HIV/AIDS, 2008–2010. Phnom Penh, National Authority for Combating Drugs and the National AIDS Authority, July 2008:12.

88. Lu F et al. Estimating the number of people at risk for and living with HIV in China in 2005: methods and results. Sexually Transmitted Infections, 2006, 82 (suppl 3): S87–S91.

89. Wang L et al. The 2007 estimates for people at risk for and living with HIV in China: progress and challenges. Journal of Acquired Immune Deficiency Syndromes, 2009, 50:414–418.

90. Xian X et al. Epidemiology of hepatitis C virus infection among injection drug users in China: systematic meta-analysis. Public Health, 2008, 122:990–1003.

91. Bao Y-P, Liu Z-M. Systematic review of HIV and HCV infection among drug users in China. International Journal of STD & AIDS, 2009, 20:399–405.

92. Reid G. HIV/AIDS among people who inject drugs in India: the current situation and national response. Presentation made at the meeting on the Development of the regional strategy for harm reduction in Asia and the Pacific 2010–2015—Confronting HIV among people who inject drugs. Kuala Lumpur, Malaysia, 7–9 December 2009.

93. National AIDS Control Organization. HIV sentinel surveillance and HIV estimation 2007: a technical brief. New Delhi, National AIDS Control Organization, Ministry of Health and Family Welfare, Government of India, October 2008.

94. Aceijas C, Rhodes T. Global estimates of prevalence of HCV infection among injecting drug users. International Journal of Drug Policy, 2007,18:352–358.

95. Phimphachanh C, Sayabounthavong K. The HIV/AIDS/STI situation in Lao's People's Republic. AIDS Education and Prevention, 2004, 16 (suppl. A):91–99.

96. UNODC ROSA. UNODC's response for prevention of HIV among drug users in South Asia through opioid substitution treatment (OST): Maldives. Accessed on 02 June 2010 at http://www.unodc.org/india/ost_interventions_scenario.html#maldives.

97. Cook C, Kanaef N. The global state of harm reduction 2008: mapping the response to drug-related HIV and hepatitis C epidemics. International Harm Reduction Association, 2008.

98. Sherstha IL. Seroprevalence of antibodies to hepatitis C virus among injecting drug users from Kathmandu. Kathmandu University Medical Journal, 2006, I:101–103.

99. Pakistan Institute of Legislative Development and Transparency. Narcotics and Pakistan: background paper. Islamabad, Pakistan, Pakistan Institute of Legislative Development and Transparency, March 2010. Accessed on 02 June 2010 from http://www.pildat.org/Publications/publication/Democracy&LegStr/Narcotics%20&%20Pakistan%20160310.

pdf.

100 Bokhari A et al. HIV risk in Karachi and Lahore, Pakistan: an emerging epidemic in injecting and commercial sex networks. International Journal of STD and AIDS, 2007, 18:486–492.

101 Canada–Pakistan HIV/AIDS Surveillance Project. HIV second generation surveillance in Pakistan. National Report Round III. Islamabad, Pakistan, National AIDS Control Programme, Ministry of Health, 2008.

102 Aceijas C et al. Estimates of injecting drug users at the national and local level in developing and transitional countries, and gender and age distribution. Sexually Transmitted Infections, 2006, 82:10–17.

103 Belimac G. Estimates of population size, HIV prevalence and number of HIV infections among IDUs, Philippines, 2000–2007. In: Situation analysis of HIV and IDU in the Philippines. Presented at the meeting on Comprehensive Training course on HIV prevention, treatment, care and support among people who inject drugs in the Philippines, Cebu City, Philippines, 2–6 March 2009.

104 May D, Agdamag D. Philippines HIV/AIDS report and HIV/ hepatitis co-infection. Paper presented at the US–Japan Joint AIDS Hepatitis Meeting Portland Oregon, 19–21 September 2009.

105 National Dangerous Drugs Control Board, Sri Lanka. Country report on the follow up to the Declaration of Commitment on HIV/AIDS (UNGASS). Reporting period January 2006–December 2007. Colombo, Sri Lanka, Ministry of Health, 2008.

106 The Asian Epidemic Model (AEM). Projections for HIV/AIDS in Thailand 2005–2025. Bangkok, Thailand, Family Health International (FHI) and the Bureau of AIDS, TB and STIs, Department of Disease Control, Ministry of Public Health, 2008.

107 Quan VM et al. Risks for HIV, HBV, and HCV infections among injection drug users in northern Vietnam: a case–control study. AIDS Care, 2009, 21:7–16.

108 Burnet Institute. HIV in the Pacific, 1984–2007. Melbourne, Australia, Burnet Institute, 2009,

109 Walmsley R. World prison population list, eighth edition. London, King's College, International Centre for Prison Studies, 2008.

110 Buavirat A et al. Risk of prevalent HIV infection associated with incarceration among injecting drug users in Bangkok, Thailand: a case–controlled study. British Medical Journal, 2003, 326:308–312.

111 UNODC/UNAIDS. Bangladesh country advocacy brief: injecting drug use and HIV. Dhaka, UN Regional Task Force on Injecting Drug Use and HIV/AIDS, October 2009. Accessed on 02 June 2010 at http://www.unodc.org/documents/eastasiaandpacific//topics/hiv-aids/UNRTF/BD_CAB_7_Oct_09_.pdf

112 The Socialist Republic of Viet Nam. The third country report on following up the implementation to the Declaration of Commitment on HIV and AIDS. Reporting period: January 2006–December 2007. Hanoi, Ministry of Health, January 2008.

113 National Authority for Combating Drugs (NACD). Report on illicit drug data and routine surveiillance systems in Cambodia 2007. Phnom Penh, Cambodia, Secretariat General

of the National Authority for Combating Drugs, Ministry of Interior, June 2008.

114   National Narcotics Control Commisssion (NNCC). Presentation at Global SMART Programme workshop, Bangkok Thailand, 29–31 June 2009.

115   National Narcotics Board (BNN) Indonesia. Improving ATS data and information systems national report. Jakarta, Indonesia, BNN Research Development and Information Centre, October 2005.

116   Doran C. An analysis of, and proposed methodology for, measuring the socio-economic impact of drugs, crime and corruption in the Lao PDR. UNODC/University of New South Wales, September 2008.

117   UNODC. Amphetamines and ecstasy. 2008 global ATS assessment. Vienna, UNODC, 2008.

118   Standing Office on Drug Control (SODC) Viet Nam. Country report by Viet Nam. 32nd meeting of heads of National

119   Drug law enforcement agencies, Asia and the Pacific, Bangkok, 10–13 February 2009.

120   Reference Group to the United Nations on HIV and injecting drug use. The global epidemiology of methamphetamine injection: a review of the evidence on use and association with HIV and other harms. Sydney, National Drug and Alcohol Research Centre, University of New South Wales, 2007. Accessed on 02 June 2010 at http://www.idurefgroup.unsw.edu.au/IDURGWeb.nsf/resources/thematic+papers/$file/methamphetamine+injecting+and+HIV+review.pdf.

121   UNAIDS. United Nations General Assembly Special Session on HIV/AIDS. Monitoring the Declaration of Commitment on HIV/AIDS: guidelines on construction of core indicators. Geneva, UNAIDS, 2002:12.

122   UNODC Commission on Narcotic Drugs. Political declaration and plan of action on international cooperation towards an integrated and balanced strategy to counter the world drug problem. Vienna, High level segment Commission on Narcotic Drugs, 11–12 March 2009. Accessed on 02 June 2010 at http://www.unodc.org/documents/commissions/CND-Uploads/CND-52-RelatedFiles/V0984963-English.pdf

123   ASEAN. Bangkok Political Declaration in pursuit of a drug-free ASEAN 2015. Bangkok, Thailand, ASEAN Secretariat, 11–13 October 2000.Accessed on 02 June 2010 at http://www.aseansec.org/5714.htm.

124   Mathers BM et al. for the 2009 Reference Group to the UN on HIV and Injecting Drug Use. HIV prevention, treatment, and care services for people who inject drugs: a systematic review of global, regional, and national coverage. The Lancet, 2010, 375:1014–1028.

125   National AIDS Control Programme consolidated data. Islamic Republic of Afghanistan, Ministry of Public Health, 2009.

126   Rabbani S. Harm reduction program in Bangladesh: progress, opportunity and challenges. Presented at the 9th ICAAP, Bali, Indonesia, 9–13 August 2009.

127   Mesquita F et al. Accelerating harm reduction interventions to confront the HIV epidemic in the Western Pacific and Asia: the role of WHO (WPRO). Harm Reduction Journal, 2008, 5:26 Accessed on 28 April 2010 at http://www.harmreductionjournal.com/content/5/1/26.

127   Wu Z. Update of harm reduction in China. In: The Second SIDA Project Advisory

Committee Meeting, Manila, the Philippines, November 2008.

128 Mboi N; Indonesian National AIDS Commission. HIV interventions for injecting drug users at multiple levels. The Indonesian experience: government and civil society partnership model for expanding coverage of harm reduction. Presented at the Symposium session on Scaling-up harm reduction services towards universal access in Asia: models of good practice. Organized by the United Nations Regional Task Force on Injecting Drug Use and HIV/AIDS for Asia and the Pacific. 9th ICAAP, Bali, Indonesia, 11 August, 2009.

129 Yuswan F; Ministry of Health, Malaysia. Scaling up harm reduction services: Malaysia's experience. Presented at the meeting on the Development of the regional strategy for harm reduction in Asia and the Pacific 2010–2015—Confronting HIV among people who inject drugs. Kuala Lumpur, Malaysia, 7–9 December, 2009.

130 National AIDS Programme. National strategic plan for HIV/AIDS in Myanmar. Progress peport 2008. Yangon, Ministry of Health, 2008.

131 Ministry of Health, Socialist Republic of Viet Nam. HIV/AIDS control and prevention for the first 6 months 2009 and working plan for the last 6 months of 2009. Hanoi, Ministry of Health, 18 September 2009.

132 International Drug Policy Consortium (IDPC). Methadone now available in Afghanistan. Alert 23 February 2010. Accessed on 02 June 2010 at http://www.idpc.net/alerts/methadone-now-available-in-afghanistan.

133 UNODC ROSA. Maldives marks the first anniversary of its ever first methadone clinic. Press release, November 2009. Accessed on 02 June 2010 at http://www.unodc.org/india/en/methadone-is-my-cure.html.

134 Sharma M et al. A situation update on HIV epidemics among people who inject drugs and national responses in South-East Asia Region. AIDS, 2009, 23:1405–1413.

135 UNODC/UNAIDS. Myanmar country advocacy brief. Injecting drug use and HIV. Myanmar, 2010. Accessed on 02 June 2010 at http://www.unodc.org/documents/eastasiaandpacific//topics/hiv-aids/UNRTF/Mya_CAB_04_Feb_10_.pdf.

136 The National Task Force on Harm Reduction, Ministry of Health of Malaysia. Final progress report. Needle and syringe exchange program pilot project. Kuala Lumpur, Ministry of Health, 2007.

137 Hammet TM et al. Law enforcement influences on HIV prevention for injection drug users: observation from a cross-border project in China and Vietnam. International Journal of Drug Policy, 2005, 16:235–245.

138 Pang LHY et al. Effectiveness of first eight methadone maintenance treatment clinics in China. AIDS, 2007, 21:103–107.

139 Ramly R. Harm reduction program in Malaysia. In: Second Sida Project Advisory Committee Meeting. Manila, Philippines, Ministry of Health, 2008.

140 Response Beyond Borders. The first Asian consultation on the prevention of HIV related to drug use. Goa, India, January 2008.